FITNESS FOR THE TIME-PRESSED

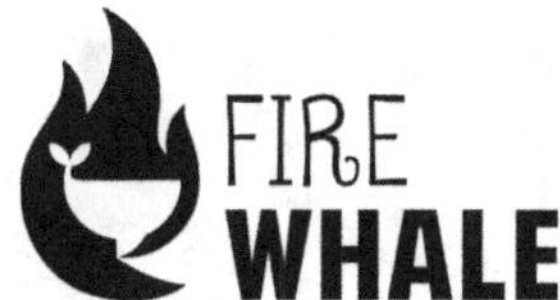

FITNESS FOR THE TIME-PRESSED

42 QUICK WORKOUTS

JASMINE WILLIAMS

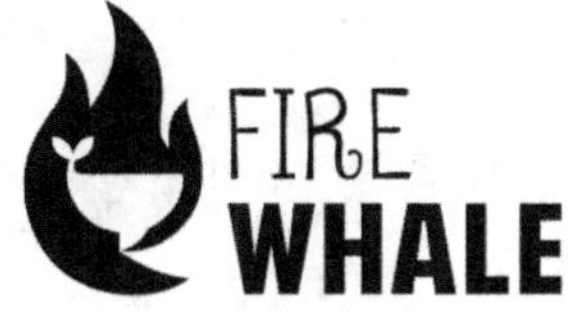

TABLE OF CONTENTS

INTRODUCTION

Welcome to "Fitness for the Time-Pressed: 42 Quick Workouts," the guidebook for squeezing health and vitality into your bustling schedule. If you've ever glanced at the clock and wondered, "How can I possibly fit exercise into my day?", you're not alone. In our fast-paced world, dedicating hours to the gym seems as archaic as a VHS tape. This book, enriched with two decades of fitness expertise and practical wisdom, is your pocket-sized personal trainer for those days when 24 hours just don't seem enough.

The 'Why' Behind Quick Workouts

Even amidst a heap of work deadlines, household chores, and a social calendar that rivals a royal tour, maintaining your health can't be negotiable. Regular exercise is the secret sauce to skyrocketing your energy levels, boosting your mood, and, of course, building a strong, resilient body. But here's the good news: long workouts aren't necessarily the key to great health. Short, but effective bursts of movement can work wonders!

Let's get straight to the point - this book isn't just about "getting it over with quickly." It's about *smart, strategic* fitness that fits snugly into your hectic life. We'll be your guide to:

- *Maximizing your time* with workouts that give you the best bang for your buck.

- *Blazing through plateaus* with high-intensity tactics.

• *Scattering seeds of exercise* throughout your day so subtly that it becomes second nature.

Proof in the Pudding – Or in This Case, the Push-Up

"How can I get fit in mere minutes?" you might ask. Let's pause and picture a busy morning that still allows for a full-body blast. You roll out of bed and while your coffee brews, you knock out a 7-minute circuit that gets your heart pumping and muscles humming. Or envision a lunch break where, instead of scrolling endlessly through your phone, you power through a brisk walk and bodyweight routine that leaves you invigorated for the afternoon. These aren't just fantasy scenarios - they're easily-attainable chapters of this book that we'll explore together.

What You'll Discover Inside

Each chapter in this book is a pearl of compact exercise elegance. They're designed to be accessible for all levels, scalable for varying intensities, and blissfully brief. Let's peek at what's ahead:

• **The 7-Minute Full Body Blast:** Think you can't set every muscle on fire in 7 minutes? Think again! This chapter will show you how.

• **Dynamic Warm-Ups:** Just a few minutes to ensure your muscles are prepped and less prone to injury – a non-negotiable for the time-crunched athlete.

• **Stairwell Workouts:** Who knew that the stairwell in your office building could be a fitness oasis? We'll explore how to make those steps count.

• And so much more – from *Office-Friendly Moves* to *Speedy Tai Chi Stretch*, every page turns with a promise of efficiency and effectiveness.

Here's the bottom line: whether it's a case of 'so much to do, so little time' or 'I'm just not the gym type,' these quick workouts are tailored to slot seamlessly into your life.

In the chapters ahead, we will lace up our metaphorical sneakers and delve into routines that are not only quick but engaging, varied, and, you guessed it – fun! Each chapter flourishes with real-life examples and illustrative anecdotes, ensuring the wisdom within is not just read, but felt and applied.

So, flip this page, and let's embark on a journey where the ticking clock is no longer a foe but a friend in your fitness odyssey. Ready, set, and let's get moving – swiftly!

THE 7-MINUTE FULL BODY BLAST

The Key Ideas

The 7-Minute Full Body Blast is a focused, time-efficient workout designed for those who wish to maximize their fitness results without spending hours at the gym. This workout combines high-intensity interval training (HIIT) with compound exercises that engage multiple muscle groups simultaneously. The aim is to elevate your heart rate and challenge your muscles, resulting in both cardiovascular and strength benefits.

• **Efficiency:** Quick bursts of intense exercise followed by brief recovery periods.

• **Accessibility:** No equipment required, suitable for all fitness levels with modifications.

• **Variety:** A range of exercises to target the whole body in one session.

• **Flexibility:** Can be performed anywhere, from your living room to a hotel room.

• **Balance:** Combines cardiovascular and strength training to promote overall fitness.

Practical Implementation

To begin, ensure your body is ready for vigorous activity with a short warm-up. Execute each exercise for 30 seconds, followed by a 10-second rest period before moving to the next exercise. Perform the sequence twice for a total of 7 minutes.

Here's your exercise line-up:

1. **Jumping Jacks:** A classic cardio move to kickstart your heart rate.

2. **Wall Sit:** Strengthens the quadriceps, glutes, and calves while challenging endurance.

3. **Push-Ups:** Works the chest, shoulders, and triceps for upper-body strength.

4. **Abdominal Crunches:** Focuses on the core for stability and toned abs.

5. **Step-Ups onto Chair:** Elevates heart rate while toning the legs and glutes.

6. **Squats:** Engages the lower body, enhancing strength and flexibility.

7. **Tricep Dips on Chair:** Targets the triceps for sculpted arms.

8. Modify as needed: Knee push-ups, seated abdominal crunches, or assisted squats.

9. Strive for full range of motion, executing each rep with precision and control.

10. Breath control is vital; exhale during the effort phase of the movement.

Consistency and Evaluation

To benefit most from the 7-Minute Full Body Blast, integrate it into your daily routine. Consistency is key to improving endurance, strength, and achieving measurable results.

Monitor Progress:

- **Frequency:** Aim for 5 days a week with 2 rest days interspersed.

- **Intensity:** Gradually increase the duration or add more sets as you grow stronger.

- **Personal milestones:** Set realistic goals and keep a journal of your workouts.

Evaluate your progress every two weeks by noting improvements such as:

- More repetitions completed in 30 seconds.

- Decreased rest times between exercises.

- Improved form and a higher range of movement.

Staying consistent and tracking your development will help you maintain motivation and see the tangible benefits of this compact, yet powerful workout program. Adjust the intensity and volume as needed to keep challenging yourself as you advance on your fitness journey.

HIIT FOR BUSY BEES: 10 MINUTES TO TRIUMPH

The Key Ideas

High-Intensity Interval Training (HIIT) compresses cardio and strength exercises into short bursts. For individuals crunched for time, this approach maximizes efficiency. HIIT's cornerstone is alternating intense activity with brief recovery periods.

- **Intensity Over Duration**: HIIT focuses on exerting maximum effort in short time frames.

- **Flexibility**: This regimen is adaptable to any fitness level. Adjust intensity accordingly.

- **Efficiency**: Science shows HIIT can achieve similar or greater benefits compared to prolonged exercise routines.

- **Metabolic Boost**: It increases your metabolic rate post-exercise, known as afterburn or EPOC (Excess Post-exercise Oxygen Consumption).

Practical Implementation

First, it's important to ensure you're medically cleared for high-intensity exercise. Once cleared, follow a structure:

1. **Warm-Up**: A 2-minute light aerobic exercise (e.g., jogging in place) prepares your body.

2. **Core HIIT Cycle**:

   ◦ 20 seconds full-intensity exercise (sprinting, jumping jacks)

   ◦ 40 seconds low-intensity exercise or rest

   ◦ Repeat this cycle for a total of 8 rounds.

3. **Cool Down**: Wind down with 2 minutes of stretching to aid recovery.

Some example exercises for the HIIT cycle:

- High knees

- Burpees

- Push-ups

- Squats

- Mountain climbers

Equipment-Free: All exercises can be performed with body weight alone.

Space-Efficient: HIIT doesn't need extensive space. A small room suffices.

Timing: Maintain precision with a timer to ensure structured intervals.

As you progress, tailor your routine:

• **Adjust Intensity**: Increase intensity by shortening rest intervals or elevating exercise difficulty.

• **Variety**: Mix in different exercises to target various muscle groups and avoid monotony.

Consistency and Evaluation

HIIT's success rests on consistent execution and tracking progress:

• **Routine**: Aim for at least 3 sessions per week.

• **Diary**: Keep an exercise diary to log workouts and reflect on improvements.

• **Physical Indicators**: Monitor changes in endurance, strength, and muscle tone.

• **Rest**: Heed your body's signals. Rest is crucial for repair and progress.

Safety Reminder: Avoid overexertion. If you feel dizzy, overly breathless, or in pain, stop immediately and seek medical advice.

Embed HIIT in your lifestyle as a sustainable, time-conscious exercise solution. This compact, potent workout method can yield substantial benefits with just 10 minutes a day.

MORNING QUICK-START: STRETCHING & ENERGIZING SEQUENCE

The Key Ideas

Incorporating a morning stretching and energizing routine can significantly enhance your physical energy and mental focus. The key lies in targeted movements that stimulate blood flow, engage your muscles, and awaken your nervous system. A series of dynamic stretches can serve as a bridge between your restful night and a productive day.

Dynamic Stretching: Dynamic stretches are active movements that take your joints and muscles through a full range of motion. This type of stretching is ideal for warming up your body and enhancing muscular performance.

Circulation: Stretching in the morning boosts circulation, delivering essential nutrients and oxygen to your muscles and brain.

Muscle Activation: Morning stretches activate your postural muscles, which can reduce the stiffness you feel after a night's rest.

Cognitive Clarity: Exercise, including stretching, releases endorphins, which contribute to a feeling of alertness and can improve mood.

Practical Implementation

1. **Cat-Cow Stretch**: Start on all fours. Inhale, arch your back, tilt your pelvis, and look up (Cow). Exhale, round your spine toward the ceiling and tuck your chin to your chest (Cat). Repeat for 1-2 minutes.

2. **Standing Forward Bend**: Stand straight, then hinge at your hips to fold forward. Let your head hang and hold elbows with opposite hands. Gently sway side to side for 1-2 minutes.

3. **Lunge with a Twist**: Step forward into a lunge. Place your opposite hand on the ground and extend the other toward the sky, rotating your torso. Hold for 15-30 seconds each side.

4. **Leg Swings**: Stand on one leg and swing the other leg forward and backward, then side to side. Do this for 30 seconds on each leg.

5. **Arm Circles**: Extend your arms sideways and perform small circles for 30 seconds, then increase to larger circles for another 30 seconds.

Finish your routine with 1 minute of deep breathing to bring oxygen to your muscles and clear the mind.

To incorporate these stretches into your routine:

- **Plan Ahead**: Set your workout clothes aside the night before.

- **Set a Reminder**: Use an app or alarm as a cue to start stretching.

- **Variation**: Keep the sequence fresh to maintain engagement and progress.

Consistency and Evaluation

Consistency in your morning routine is key for long-term benefits.
Track your regularity and note how your body responds. Adjust
the sequence duration and intensity as needed.

Reflect on your energy levels and mental clarity post-routine to
evaluate effectiveness. Tweak the sequence based on personal
needs. Remember, it's not just about flexibility but overall well-
being.

A successful morning stretching and energizing sequence should
leave you feeling activated, not exhausted. It should harmonize
with your life, improve your day-to-day function, and support your
time management goals by seamlessly integrating into your
morning.

LUNCH BREAK POWER WALK & TONE-UP

The Key Ideas

Maximizing your lunch break for fitness means understanding the concept of incidental exercise—integrating movement into your routine not designated as a formal workout. The power walk and tone-up session combines cardiovascular health with strength training in a time-efficient manner. Here's what you need to know:

- **Effective Time Management**: Your lunch break is precious, and every minute counts. A planned power walk allows for cardiovascular benefits within a constrained timeframe.

- **Incorporating Strength Moves**: Scatter bodyweight exercises during the walk to hit major muscle groups without needing a gym.

- **No Special Equipment Needed**: Save time and hassle. You just need comfortable clothing and supportive shoes.

- **Mind and Body Refresh**: This midday activity can boost mental clarity and combat afternoon fatigue.

Practical Implementation

Implement this workout with the following steps:

1. **Plan Your Route**: Before your break, have a clear path mapped out. This avoids wasting time deciding where to go.

2. **Dress Appropriately**: Wear or bring clothes and shoes suitable for walking and light exercises.

3. **Warm-Up**: Spend 3-5 minutes stretching to limber up and prevent injuries.

4. **Power Walk**: Start your walk at a brisk pace. Your heart rate should rise, and you should be able to talk but not sing.

5. **Strength Exercises**: Every 5 minutes, stop to do a one-minute set of exercises like squats, lunges, push-ups, or tricep dips.

6. **Cool Down**: Slow your pace in the last 5 minutes and end with stretching to reduce muscle soreness.

7. **Stay Hydrated**: Drink water before, during, and after to stay hydrated.

Consistency and Evaluation

- **Track Progress**: Log your walks and exercises daily. Notice changes in endurance and strength over time.

- **Seek Variety**: Change your route and exercises to work different muscles and prevent boredom.

- **Evaluate Frequency**: Aim for at least three power walk and tone-ups per week.

- **Adjust Intensity**: As you get fitter, increase the speed of your walk and the intensity of the strength exercises.

- **Listen to Your Body**: Rest when necessary. Balance is key to avoiding burnout or injury.

Implementing this routine is a straightforward way to integrate fitness into your busy schedule. Stay consistent, and you'll reap the benefits.

5-MINUTE DESKERCISE: OFFICE-FRIENDLY MOVES

The Key Ideas

Sitting for prolonged periods is detrimental to your health. Integrate movement into your workday to combat the effects of a sedentary lifestyle. Deskercise comprises quick, simple exercises that can be performed at or near your desk, requiring minimal space. These movements improve circulation, reduce tension, and increase focus.

Practical Implementation

- **Chair Squats**: Stand up from your chair, lower your body back down, stopping right before you sit back down. Do 10 reps.

- **Desk Push-Ups**: Place hands on the edge of your desk, walk your feet out to a 45-degree angle, and perform push-ups. Complete 10-15 reps.

- **Shoulder Shrugs**: Raise both shoulders up to your ears, hold for 1-2 seconds, and relax. Repeat for 8-10 reps.

- **Seated Leg Lifts**: While seated, keep your feet flat on the floor, straighten one leg, and hold in place for a few seconds. Lower back down without touching the floor and repeat 10 times. Switch legs.

• **Desk Chair Swivels**: Sit upright and lift your feet slightly off the ground. Hold the edge of your desk and use your core to swivel the chair from side to side. Do 15 swivels.

• **Arm Circles**: Extend your arms out to the sides and do small, controlled circles for 20-30 seconds in each direction.

• **Neck Rolls**: Relax your neck, lower your chin to your chest, and slowly roll your head in a circular motion. Do 3 rotations each side.

Reminder

• Use smooth motions; don't jerk or rush.

• Avoid holding your breath; keep breathing steadily.

• Tailor the reps based on your comfort level.

Consistency and Evaluation

To gain benefits, integrate these exercises into your routine at least once every hour. Track your consistency with a simple log or a mobile app. Evaluate how you feel after a week—note increases in alertness, reduced stiffness, and improved mood. Adjust the frequency and intensity as needed. Networks and accountability can enhance consistency, so consider a deskercise buddy or group to stay motivated.

DYNAMIC WARM-UPS: 3 MINUTES TO ACTIVATED MUSCLES

The Key Ideas

Warm-ups matter. A dynamic warm-up prepares not just muscles, but also your nervous system, for the workout ahead.

- **Elevated Heart Rate**: Increases blood flow, enhancing the delivery of oxygen and nutrients.

- **Muscle Temperature**: Warmed muscles exhibit greater flexibility and efficiency.

- **Joint Mobility**: Movement lubricates joints, reducing the risk of injury.

- **Mental Preparedness**: Establishes a workout mindset for focus and performance.

Key Idea: Quick, effective dynamic warm-ups are crucial for a safe and effective workout, especially when time is scarce.

Practical Implementation

Strategy Is Key: A smart approach ensures you cover all muscle groups swiftly.

- **Upper Body Activation**:

  1. Arm Circles – 20 seconds

  2. Shoulder Shrugs – 20 seconds

  3. Torso Twists – 20 seconds

- **Lower Body Activation**:

  1. Leg Swings – 20 seconds each leg

  2. Hip Rotations – 20 seconds each direction

  3. Ankle Rolls – 20 seconds each ankle

- **Core Activation**:

  1. Standing Bicycle Crunches – 30 seconds

  2. Invisible Jump Rope – 30 seconds

- **Overall Dynamic Stretch**: High Knees or Butt Kicks - 30 seconds

Key Idea: Tailor the warm-up to your day's workout, focusing on the specific muscle groups you'll be using.

Consistency and Evaluation

Track and Adapt: Monitor how your body responds.

- **Consistency**: Commit to three minutes before each workout, without exception.

- **Variety**: Change your warm-up routines periodically to keep them fresh and comprehensive.

• **Assess Effectiveness**: Are you experiencing fewer injuries? Better workout performance?

• **Tweak As Necessary**: Adjust the time spent on each exercise based on your body's feedback.

Key Idea: Regular evaluation of your warm-up's effectiveness is crucial to maintaining its benefits over time.

INTENSE ABS SESSION: 6 MINUTES TO A STRONGER CORE

The Key Ideas

Your core is the powerhouse of your body. A strong core aids in stability, posture, and overall strength. Six minutes is all it takes each day to target and enhance your abdominal muscles. This chapter focuses on maximizing workout efficiency with targeted exercises for rapid core development.

• Quick Workouts: Time is precious; intensity over duration yields results.

• Exercise Selection: Simple yet powerful movements that engage the entire core.

• Progression: Gradually increasing intensity to challenge muscles.

• Recovery: Importance of allowing muscles to heal for growth.

• Technique: Precision over speed to maximize gains and reduce injury risk.

Practical Implementation

The Workout Plan:

1. **Plank:** 1 minute

   ○ Form straight line from shoulders to heels.

   ○ Engage core, squeeze glutes.

2. **Russian Twists:** 1 minute

   ○ Feet off ground, twist torso side to side.

   ○ Touch hands to the floor each side.

3. **Side Planks:** 30 seconds each side

   ○ Stack feet, lift hips, extend arm upwards.

   ○ Keep body in straight line.

4. **Bicycle Crunches:** 1 minute

   ○ Touch opposite elbow to knee, alternate sides.

   ○ Extend the other leg fully.

5. **Leg Raises:** 1 minute

   ○ Lying down, lift legs straight up, lower without touching floor.

   ○ Hands under buttocks for support.

6. **Mountain Climbers:** 1 minute

   ○ In plank, drive knees to chest alternately.

   ○ Maintain a brisk pace.

Key Points:

- Perform each exercise back-to-back with minimal rest.

- Control your movements to prevent momentum cheating.

- Modify exercises to suit your fitness level.

- Focus on form to reduce injury risk and maximize efficiency.

Equipment:

No equipment is necessary, making this workout accessible and convenient.

Timing:

- First thing in the morning or during any spare six-minute block.

- Set a timer to keep track of each minute.

Consistency and Evaluation

Consistency: Core strength requires consistent effort. Aim for this six-minute session daily to see measurable improvements.

- Track your sessions.

- Aim for gradual increase in exercise difficulty.

Evaluation:

- Weekly self-assessment of firmness and strength in your midsection.

- Monthly progress check through increased reps or hold times.

To summarize, unlocking a stronger core doesn't require hours at the gym. A high-intensity, focused six-minute session can effectively boost core strength if performed consistently with proper form. Remember, this is a starting point; adjust the intensity as you progress to continue challenging your muscles. Regular evaluation will guide your advancement and maintain motivation. Stay diligent, and a stronger core will follow.

ULTIMATE PUSH-UP CHALLENGE: VARIATIONS IN 5 MINUTES

The Key Ideas

- **Essentials First**: Understand the proper form of a traditional push-up.

- **Variety is Key**: Incorporate different push-up variations to target various muscle groups.

- **Timed Challenge**: Perform each variation for 1 minute, aiming for quality over quantity.

- **Progressive Overload**: Gradually increase difficulty to continue muscle growth and strength.

- **Rest and Recovery**: Allow brief rest periods between variations to maintain form and prevent injury.

Practical Implementation

1. **Traditional Push-Up**: Start in a plank position with hands under shoulders. Lower your body until your chest nearly touches the floor. Push up to the starting position. Aim for maximum reps with perfect form for 1 minute.

2. **Incline Push-Up**: Place your hands on a raised surface—like a bench or step. Perform push-ups with your body at a slight incline. This variation puts less strain on the shoulders.

3. **Decline Push-Up**: Elevate your feet using a bench or step. With hands on the ground, perform a push-up. This targets the upper chest and shoulders.

4. **Diamond Push-Up**: Bring your hands together under your chest to form a diamond shape with your fingers. Lower and lift, focusing on triceps engagement.

5. **Wide-Grip Push-Up**: Position your hands wider than shoulder-width. Lower your body, emphasizing the pectoral muscles.

6. **Cool Down**: Stretch your chest, shoulders, and arms to aid in recovery.

Consistency and Evaluation

• **Daily Challenge**: Incorporate these variations into a daily routine.

• **Record Keeping**: Track the number of repetitions completed in each 1-minute interval to measure progress.

• **Listen to Your Body**: If an exercise causes pain, stop immediately and consider consulting a fitness professional.

• **Adjust Intensity**: If the challenge becomes too easy, add repetitions or decrease rest time to maintain intensity.

STAIRWELL WORKOUTS: CLIMBING TO FITNESS IN NO TIME

The Key Ideas

Stairwell workouts offer an effective way to harness the essence of cardio and strength training combined. Here's why they're impactful:

- **Accessibility**: Most buildings have a set of stairs available.

- **Efficiency**: Stair climbing engages multiple muscle groups, offering a comprehensive workout.

- **Adaptable Intensity**: You can alter the intensity to suit fitness levels and goals.

- **No Equipment Necessary**: Eliminates the need for a gym subscription or purchasing equipment.

Essential benefits include improved cardiovascular health, enhanced muscle tone, and increased calorie burn, which can support weight management.

Practical Implementation

To make stairwell workouts part of your routine, follow these steps:

1. **Safety First**: Ensure the stairwell is well-lit, has sturdy railings, and the steps are not slippery.

2. **Warm-up**: Start with 5 minutes of light cardio, like jogging in place or walking up and down one flight.

3. **The Workout**:

   - Begin with a single flight climb, walking briskly. This is your baseline.

   - Progress to running up the stairs for a higher intensity burst.

   - Increase the challenge by taking two steps at a time, to target glute and leg muscles more intensely.

   - Introduce lateral steps or stair hops for added variety.

4. **Cool Down**: Finish with a slow descent and gentle stretching of all major muscle groups used.

For a structured program, consider:

- Short workouts: 1-minute stair runs, 30-second rest, repeat for 10-15 minutes.

- Long workouts: Climbing for 20-30 minutes at a steady pace, 2-3 times a week.

Consistency and Evaluation

Consistency is crucial. Aim to integrate stairwell workouts into your schedule at least twice a week. Tracking progress is key:

- Time your stair climbs and aim to reduce this over successive workouts.

- Count how many flights you can climb before fatigue sets in and work to increase this number.

- Note improvements in general fitness levels, such as reduced heart rate after climbing or quicker recovery time.

Evaluate your routine every 4 weeks and adjust as necessary to continue challenging your body and seeing results. Remember, it isn't about the speed or the number of stairs climbed, but the commitment to enhancing your fitness through consistent, intentional actions.

YOGA FLOW FOR FOCUS: 12 MINUTES OF SERENITY

The Key Ideas

You have twelve minutes. Perhaps between meetings, after dropping off the kids, or in that short window before your day ramps up. These twelve mindful minutes can drastically enhance your focus and clarity. Let's dissect the Yoga Flow for Focus, a sequence designed to align your body and mind.

Yoga is a practice steeped in both physical and mental discipline. It strengthens, it stretches, and it stabilizes. But for many, its most treasured gift is the cultivation of serenity and sharp focus. The routine we'll explore can reset your mental state, propelling you into heightened awareness and productivity.

This flow centers on poses known for their focus-enhancing properties. Each asana is a building block towards mental clarity.

Practical Implementation

Begin in a comfortable, distraction-free space. Lay out your yoga mat or find a soft surface. Dress in flexible attire. Here's your flow:

1. **Mountain Pose (Tadasana)**: Stand tall with feet together. Breathe deeply, grounding yourself.

2. **Tree Pose (Vrksasana)**: Balance on one foot, the other foot resting on the opposing thigh. Find a focal point and breathe.

3. **Eagle Pose (Garudasana)**: Twist your legs and arms into one another. Squat slightly. Concentrate on maintaining balance.

4. **Standing Forward Bend (Uttanasana)**: Hinge at the hips, fold forward. Let your head hang, releasing neck tension.

5. **Downward-Facing Dog (Adho Mukha Svanasana)**: Form a triangle with your body, hands, and feet pressing down, hips high.

6. **Warrior II (Virabhadrasana II)**: Step into a lunge, back foot at a 90-degree angle. Arms reach out, gaze over front hand.

7. **Extended Triangle Pose (Utthita Trikonasana)**: Straighten the front leg, reach forward, then tilt into a triangle formation.

8. **Seated Forward Bend (Paschimottanasana)**: Sitting, stretch legs forward, fold over them, reaching for your toes.

9. **Child's Pose (Balasana)**: Kneel, then fold forward, forehead to the ground, arms extended.

Repeat these poses in a smooth, unhurried sequence. Focus on your breath; it's the rhythmic guide for your movement and stillness. Allow the inhalations and exhalations to grow deeper as you progress through the routine. Each pose should be held for five to six breaths, or longer if your schedule allows.

Consistency and Evaluation

Incorporating this flow into your daily routine is where the true value emerges. Consistent practice fortifies focus. Reflect after each session. Have your thoughts slowed? Is there a presence of calm? Mark these observations.

Set a regular time for this routine. Morning, to awaken and focus for the day, or afternoon, to reset. Make your practice non-negotiable, akin to brushing your teeth. Over time, evaluate its impact:

- Has your concentration improved?

- Do tasks seem less daunting?

- Is there an increase in your productivity?

Adjust the practice as needed. The beauty of yoga lies in its flexibility and personal adaptation.

Remember, focus is not simply granted; it's cultivated. Through your twelve-minute Yoga Flow for Focus, harness a quieter mind, a sharper focus, and embrace serenity in your daily rush.

RESISTANCE BAND BLITZ: FULL BODY IN 10 MINUTES

The Key Ideas

Exercise doesn't need to be time-consuming to be effective. A resistance band—a lightweight, portable tool—facilitates a high-intensity workout for your whole body within just ten minutes. Embrace the following concepts:

- **Efficiency**: Target multiple muscle groups simultaneously.

- **Intensity**: Work at a high level of exertion to maximize the short time frame.

- **Progression**: Increase resistance and complexity over time to continue improvements.

- **Flexibility**: Adapt exercises according to your space and circumstances.

Practical Implementation

Warm-Up (1 Minute)

1. Arm Circles: 30 seconds forward and backward movements.

2. Leg Swings: 30 seconds each leg, forward and side-to-side motions.

Exercise Routine (8 Minutes)

1. **Squats with Overhead Press**

   ○ Stand on the band with feet shoulder-width apart.

   ○ Hold the ends and squat; as you rise, press your arms overhead.

   ○ Perform for 1 minute.

2. **Chest Press**

   ○ Anchor the band behind you at chest level.

   ○ Face away, press the band forward explosively, and slowly return.

   ○ Continue for 1 minute.

3. **Bent-Over Rows**

   ○ Stand on the band, hinge at the waist.

   ○ Pull the band towards your waist, then release with control.

   ○ Repeat for 1 minute.

4. **Standing Lateral Leg Lifts**

   ○ Place band around ankles.

   ○ Lift leg to the side against the resistance, switch after 30 seconds.

5. **Core Twists**

   ○ Sit with legs slightly bent, band around the feet.

   ○ Hold band with both hands, twist torso side to side.

   ○ Engage for 1 minute.

6. **Bicep Curls**

   - Stand on the band, elbows stationary.

   - Curl hands toward shoulders, then extend with control.

   - Commit to 1 minute.

7. **Triceps Extension**

   - Anchor the band overhead.

   - Pull down, keeping elbows fixed and close to head.

   - Continue for 1 minute.

8. **Plank Pull**

   - In a plank position, place the band under one hand.

   - Pull the band up with the opposite hand, keeping your body stable.

   - Alternate sides for 1 minute.

Cool-Down (1 Minute)

1. *Shoulder Stretch*: Hold the band with both hands, arms extended, raise over and behind the head.

2. *Hamstring Stretch*: Sit and loop the band over one foot, pull gently towards yourself, switch after 30 seconds.

Consistency and Evaluation

Commit to this 10-minute full-body blitz daily. Track your performance:

- **Endurance**: Can you sustain each exercise for the full duration?

• **Strength**: Are the resistance levels still challenging you?

• **Form**: Maintain proper technique throughout each movement.

Progress by increasing resistance band strength, or adding complexity with compound movements. This quick, dynamic sequence eschews excuses and ensures you can fit fitness into your daily routine. Complete regimens yield results; consistency trumps all. Adjust as needed but maintain the rhythm of your routine for long-term benefits.

CALISTHENICS QUICK CIRCUIT: STRENGTH WITHOUT EQUIPMENT

The Key Ideas

- **Calisthenics** utilizes gravity and body weight for resistance training.

- **Efficiency** is paramount; a circuit approach maximizes time.

- **Progression** through increased intensity or variations maintains challenge.

- A **no-equipment** routine ensures accessibility and convenience.

- **Quick circuits** achieve strength gains in a short time frame.

Practical Implementation

- **Warm-Up**: Begin with a 5-minute warm-up to get blood flowing.

  - Examples: Jumping jacks, arm circles, gentle jogging in place.

• **Exercises**: Perform each exercise for 30 seconds or 12-15 reps; rest minimally between exercises.

  1. **Push-Ups**: Standard, diamond, or wide-grip to work different muscles.

  2. **Squats**: Keep weight in heels and back straight.

  3. **Lunges**: Step forward and lower hips, then switch legs.

  4. **Dips**: Utilize a chair or low table for triceps dips.

  5. **Plank**: Elbow or extended arm plank for core conditioning.

  6. **Burpees**: Full-body exercise for endurance and power.

• **Sequence**: Run through the exercises in order, then repeat the circuit 2-3 times.

• **Modification**: Adjust each exercise to match fitness level.

  ○ Easier: Modify push-ups on knees, reduce squat depth, step back lunges.

  ○ Harder: Elevate feet for push-ups, jump squats, jump lunges.

Consistency and Evaluation

• **Routine**: Aim for at least 3 circuits a week for optimal results.

• **Progress Tracking**: Note improvements in reps, form, or reduced rest times.

• **Listen to Your Body**: Rest as needed but push for consistent progression.

• **Evaluation**: After 4 weeks, assess strength gains through increased ease of exercises or ability to perform more challenging variations.

QUICK CARDIO DRILLS: JUMP ROPE JOURNEYS

The Key Ideas

Remember the simple rope from your childhood? It's now your fitness ally. A jump rope can crank up your heart rate, enhance agility, and improve your cardiovascular fitness. Here's the raw truth: jump rope is a high-intensity exercise that targets your full body while being light on equipment and heavy on results.

- **Full-Body Workout**: Engages legs for jumping, core for stability, and arms and shoulders for turning the rope.

- **Portability**: A jump rope fits in your backpack, making it an accessible workout option anywhere.

- **Versatility**: You can change your workout intensity and style quickly, from high knees to double unders.

- **Efficient**: Gives you an intense workout in a short span of time, perfect for busy schedules.

Practical Implementation

Getting Started:

1. Choose a rope suitably sized for your height.

2. Find a space with high ceilings and a flat, non-slippery surface.

3. Wear supportive footwear for impact absorption.

Basic Drills:

4. **Single Jumps**: Start with the classic one-jump per rope turn to find your rhythm.

5. **High Knees**: Increase intensity by bringing knees higher as you jump.

6. **Boxer Step**: Shift weight from one foot to the other, mimicking a boxer's shuffle.

Advanced Movements:

• **Double Unders**: The rope passes twice per jump, rapidly increasing your heart rate.

• **Criss-Cross**: Cross your arms on alternate jumps for added upper body engagement.

• **Side Swings**: Swing the rope at your sides in between jumps to introduce an active rest period.

Remember to start with short intervals, gradually building as your stamina increases.

Sample Routine *(30 seconds per exercise, 15 seconds rest)*:

1. Single Jumps

2. High Knees

3. Boxer Step

4. Double Unders

5. Criss-Cross

6. Side Swings

7. Rest & Repeat for 3-5 rounds

Consistency and Evaluation

Like any workout, consistency trumps sporadic bursts of enthusiasm. Aim for jump rope sessions three to four times weekly, gauging progress by the ease of completing routines, increased endurance, and improving coordination.

Track Your Progress:

- **Time**: Begin with short sessions, increasing as your fitness improves.

- **Form**: Self-record or use a mirror to check form and make corrections.

- **Frequency**: Strive to reduce rest intervals between exercises.

Self-Checks:

- Notice a reduction in heart rate during rest periods.

- Experience a feeling of increased energy levels post-workout.

- Watch for improved skill execution and fewer trip-ups.

Jump rope transcends being a mere child's play to a substantial fitness journey. Pick up your rope, it's time to leap towards your health goals.

15-MINUTE FLASH DUMBBELL DRILL

The Key Ideas

Your time is precious, yet so is your health. The 15-Minute Flash Dumbbell Drill is designed to maximize your fitness within a minimal time frame. This high-intensity workout combines strength, endurance, and flexibility, targeting all major muscle groups. The key is to maintain form while pushing the pace, ensuring effectiveness without injury.

- **Intensity Over Duration**: Short bursts of high-intensity exercise can be as effective as longer workouts.

- **Compound Movements**: Engage multiple joints and muscle groups to maximize calorie burn and efficiency.

- **Minimal Equipment**: Dumbbells are versatile, portable, and accessible tools for a comprehensive workout.

- **Adaptability**: Suitable for all fitness levels with adjustable weights and intensity.

This drill's beauty lies in its simplicity, requiring just a set of dumbbells and a little space.

Practical Implementation

1. **Warm-Up (2 minutes)**

   ○ March in place with high knees.

   ○ Arm circles—forward and backward.

   ○ Leg swings—side to side and front to back.

2. **Workout Protocol (12 minutes)**

   ○ Perform each exercise for 1 minute, then immediately transition to the next.

   ○ Rest for 15 seconds between exercises if necessary.

Exercise Circuit: 1. **Squat Press** - Stand, feet shoulder-width apart, dumbbells at shoulders. - Squat down, keep your back straight. Stand and press dumbbells overhead. 2. **Dumbbell Row** - Bend forward, slight bend in knees, back flat. - Pull dumbbells towards chest, squeeze shoulder blades. 3. **Lunges with Bicep Curl** - Step forward into a lunge, dumbbells by your side. - Lower into the lunge, curl dumbbells to shoulders. 4. **Deadlift to Upright Row** - Stand with feet hip-width, dumbbells in front. - Hinge forward, flat back, then rise and pull dumbbells to chest. 5. **Dumbbell Chest Press** - Lie on the ground, knees bent, press dumbbells up from chest. 6. **Russian Twists** - Sit, lean back, knees bent, twist holding a single dumbbell.

3. Repeat the circuit for the remaining time.

4. **Cool Down (1 minute)**

   ○ Shoulder stretches—pull arm across body.

   ○ Quad stretches—hold foot to buttock, stand straight.

   ○ Hamstring stretches—reach for toes, legs straight.

Keep transitions quick to maintain elevated heart rate.

Consistency and Evaluation

Track Progress: Note the weights used, and number of sets and reps completed. As strength and endurance improve, increase weight or pace, not workout length.

Consistency Is Key: Commit to the 15-Minute Flash Dumbbell Drill 3 times per week for optimal results.

Self-Evaluation: Regularly assess your form, intensity, and recovery. If exercises become easier, it's time to progress. Feeling unduly exhausted? Scale back and re-evaluate your nutrition and rest.

Follow this simple, no-nonsense approach, and fitness can become an integrated, non-negotiable part of your busy life. With this drill, it's not about having time; it's about making time.

PLYOMETRIC POWER: EXPLOSIVE MOVES IN MINUTES

The Key Ideas

Plyometric training harnesses the power of explosive movements to enhance muscular power, speed, and endurance, all while maximizing calorie burn in a short time span.

- **Defining Plyometrics**: Repeated rapid stretching and contracting of muscles to increase muscle power.

- **Benefits**: Amplifies strength, agility, and energy. Key for sports performance; useful for everyday activities.

- **Time Efficiency**: Plyometric exercises can be executed in high-intensity bursts; ideal for quick workouts.

Practical Implementation

Begin your plyometric journey with a straightforward routine:

1. **Warm-Up**: Essential to prevent injuries. Spend 5-10 minutes on dynamic stretches or light cardio.

2. **Safety First**: Start slow, focus on form, and wear appropriate gear. Gradually increase intensity.

Sample Plyometric Session

- **Jump Squats (3 sets x 15 reps)**: Stand with feet shoulder-width apart, squat down, then explode upwards.

- **Burpees (3 sets x 10 reps)**: Squat, place hands on the floor, jump back into a plank, return to squat, then jump up.

- **Box Jumps (3 sets x 10 reps)**: Stand in front of a sturdy box, jump onto it with both feet, then step back down.

- **Plyo Push-Ups (3 sets x 10 reps)**: Perform a push-up, but push up with enough force that your hands leave the ground.

- **Skater Jumps (3 sets x 20 reps)**: Leap side-to-side, landing on one foot, imitating a speed skater.

Remember, you can modify these exercises to suit your fitness level.

Rest Intervals: Keep them short (30-60 seconds) to maintain intensity and enhance conditioning.

Consistency and Evaluation

Evaluate your performance regularly.

- Progress can be measured by the number of reps, the height of jumps, or the reduction in rest periods.

- Push for consistency in your routine. Aim for 2-3 sessions per week.

- Keep a workout log. Track exercises, repetitions, and rest periods to gauge improvement.

- Listen to your body. Adequate rest is crucial for recovery.

By integrating these explosive exercises into your routine, you will unlock a new dimension of fitness that can be achieved efficiently and effectively.

SPEEDY PILATES ROUTINE FOR CORE AND FLEXIBILITY

The Key Ideas

- **Efficiency in Movement**: Pilates exercises that target multiple muscle groups simultaneously, maximizing your workout and minimizing time spent.

- **Core Strength**: Emphasize movements focusing on the powerhouse of your body—the core—as it supports all other exercises for enhanced performance and injury prevention.

- **Flexibility Gains**: Incorporate stretches within the routine to improve joint range of motion and muscle elasticity.

- **Breath Integration**: Utilize the Pilates principle of controlled breathing to increase the effectiveness of each exercise and maintain rhythmic flow.

Practical Implementation

1. **Warm-Up**: Begin with a 5-minute dynamic stretching sequence to prepare your muscles and joints.

   - Arm sweeps

   - Leg swings

- Gentle twists

2. **The Hundred**: Start lying on your back, legs in tabletop position, and pump your arms vigorously for 100 counts. Inhale for five pumps, exhale for five.

3. **Roll-Up**: Perform a slow-motion sit-up, articulating each vertebrae, to stretch the spine and engage the abs. Do 6-8 repetitions.

4. **Single Leg Circles**: Keep one leg extended towards the ceiling and circle it clockwise then counterclockwise for 10 repetitions each before switching legs.

5. **Criss-Cross**: Bring your opposite shoulder to your knee in a twisting motion to work the obliques. Repeat 10 times on each side.

6. **Plank Series**:

   - Classic Plank: Hold for 30 seconds.

   - Side Plank: Switch sides after 15 seconds each.

   - Dynamic Plank: Engage by adding leg raises, 5 each leg.

7. **Single Leg Stretch**: Alternating leg pulls while keeping your head and shoulders lifted. Engage your abdominal muscles with each switch.

8. **Double Leg Stretch**: Extend both arms and legs from a curled position and circle arms back to hug knees. Six repetitions.

9. **Spine Stretch Forward**: Sit tall, legs extended; exhale, stretch your arms, and reach forward. Repeat this stretch 4 times.

10. **Saw**: Twist and then stretch forward toward your opposite foot. This works both flexibility and core strength.

11. **Pilates Push-Up**: A narrow stance push-up focusing on triceps strength and core stability. Perform 3-5 repetitions.

12. **Cool-Down**: End with 5 minutes of static stretching focusing on the muscles you've just worked.

- ○ Forward fold

- ○ Butterfly stretch

- ○ Spinal twist

Consistency and Evaluation

- **Regular Practice**: Aim to complete this routine at least three times a week for noticeable improvement in strength and flexibility.

- **Progress Tracking**: Note your initial flexibility, strength levels, and emotional state before starting and periodically review changes.

- **Modify as Needed**: Tailor exercises to your comfort level, ensuring proper form is prioritized over speed or range of motion.

- **Seek Feedback**: If possible, attend a session with a certified Pilates instructor for critique on your form and technique.

By dedicating 20 minutes a day to this streamlined Pilates routine, you will soon experience a stronger core, enhanced flexibility, and greater overall body awareness. Remember, the most effective workout is one that is consistent and well-executed. Persevere, and the results will follow.

TABATA TORCH: 4-MINUTE FAT-BURNING WORKOUT

The Key Ideas

Tabata training is a high-intensity interval training (HIIT) workout featuring exercises that last four minutes. It was developed by Dr. Izumi Tabata in the 1990s, originally to train Olympic speedskaters. The basic structure of the program is as follows:

- **Workout Intensity:** Perform each exercise at a very high intensity for 20 seconds.

- **Rest Period:** Rest for 10 seconds.

- **Cycle Repetition:** Complete 8 rounds of each exercise.

The key to Tabata is to push yourself to your maximum effort during the high-intensity bursts. This approach has several benefits:

- **Efficient Fat Burning:** Increases your metabolism and enhances fat burning.

- **Time-Saving:** Offers a quick workout option for those with tight schedules.

- **Increased Aerobic and Anaerobic Capacity:** Improves both cardiovascular and muscular endurance.

• **Adaptability:** Can be applied to various exercises, including sprinting, cycling, jumping, and bodyweight movements.

• **Minimal Equipment Needed:** Most Tabata exercises can be done with no equipment or whatever is handy, like a chair or wall.

Practical Implementation

To start your Tabata workout, choose four exercises that target different muscle groups for balance. Here's a simple plan:

1. **Push-ups:** Work the chest, shoulders, and triceps.

2. **Squats:** Engage the quadriceps, hamstrings, and glutes.

3. **Mountain Climbers:** Target your core and increase your heart rate.

4. **Lunges:** Focus on leg and core strength.

Tabata Torch Routine:

Perform each exercise for 20 seconds at maximum effort, then rest for 10 seconds. Move to the next exercise after each cycle. Complete two cycles of the following routine:

1. Push-ups (20s) - Rest (10s)

2. Squats (20s) - Rest (10s)

3. Mountain Climbers (20s) - Rest (10s)

4. Lunges (20s) - Rest (10s)

Repeat once more for a total of 4 minutes.

Tips for Maximum Efficiency:

• Warm-up adequately before starting your Tabata session to prevent injuries.

- Use a timer to keep track of your intervals.

- Focus on maintaining proper form, especially as you fatigue.

- Cool down and stretch post-workout to aid recovery.

Consistency and Evaluation

- **Regular Practice:** Aim to incorporate Tabata Torch into your workout regimen 3-4 times a week.

- **Progress Tracking:** Keep a log of reps or distance for each exercise to track improvements.

- **Intensity Adjustment:** As your fitness improves, up the intensity or incorporate weights.

- **Recovery:** Allow for at least one day of rest between Tabata sessions to prevent overtraining.

- **Health Monitor:** Listen to your body and adjust as needed, especially if you're feeling undue strain or pain.

Success Markers:

- Increased rep count over time.

- Improved recovery rate after sessions.

- Enhanced overall endurance and stamina.

- Noticeable fat loss when combined with a balanced diet.

By adhering to these principles, you can maximize the benefits of Tabata Torch. Stick with it, and you'll soon reap the rewards of this condensed yet potent workout format.

CHAIR WORKOUTS: SEATED EXERCISE SERIES

The Key Ideas

Chair workouts provide a flexible and accessible method to stay active. These exercises are designed for efficiency, targeting multiple muscle groups while seated. Here are the key ideas:

- **Accessibility:** Chair exercises can be performed anywhere with a sturdy chair, making it perfect for those with limited mobility or space.

- **Safety:** A seated position reduces the risk of falls, making it ideal for all fitness levels, especially beginners or those with balance concerns.

- **Versatility:** A wide range of exercises can be adapted to a seated position, working every major muscle group in the body.

- **Integration:** These workouts can be seamlessly incorporated into daily routines, like during a lunch break or while watching TV.

Practical Implementation

To get started with chair workouts, follow this step-by-step guide. Remember, begin each workout with a warm-up and conclude with a cool-down.

1. **Warm-Up**

   ○ Shoulder rolls: Lift your shoulders up, roll them back, and then down in a circular motion.

   ○ Ankle circles: Lift your foot off the ground and rotate your ankle in a circular motion.

2. **Upper Body**

   ○ Arm circles: Extend arms out to the sides and rotate in small and large circles.

   ○ Bicep curls: Use water bottles or cans as weights, bend the elbow to lift towards the shoulder.

   ○ Tricep dips: Hands on the edge of the seat, slide off and bend elbows to lower body, then push up.

3. **Core**

   ○ Seated twists: Keep feet flat on the ground while twisting the torso from side to side.

   ○ Chair planks: Place hands on the seat and extend your body into a plank position.

4. **Lower Body**

   ○ Seated leg lifts: Lift one leg at a time, keeping it straight, hold, then lower.

   ○ Knee extensions: Extend one leg out straight, hold, then lower the foot back to the floor.

5. **Flexibility**

   ◦ Overhead stretch: Extend arms above the head, interlace fingers, and lean from side to side.

   ◦ Seated pigeon: Place one foot over the opposite knee and lean forward for a hip stretch.

6. **Cool-Down**

   ◦ Deep breathing: Sit back comfortably, close your eyes, and take slow, deep breaths.

   ◦ Neck stretches: Tilt your head from side to side, then look down and up to relax neck muscles.

Consistency and Evaluation

Develop a routine and stick to it. Consistency is key to gain benefits from chair workouts. Track progress by noting increases in repetitions, improved flexibility, or enhanced comfort when performing daily activities.

- **Routine:** Aim for a minimum of three sessions per week.

- **Adaptation:** As strength builds, increase the difficulty by adding weights or extending the duration of exercises.

- **Assessment:** Every few weeks, evaluate your comfort level and adjust your workout accordingly.

Remember, the best workout is the one you do regularly. Chair workouts offer a practical approach to fitness that fits any schedule and space, without compromising effectiveness. Stay committed, evaluate your progress, and enjoy the journey towards better health.

BATHROOM BODYWEIGHT BONANZA: TINY SPACE FITNESS

The Key Ideas

Exercising within the limited confines of a bathroom necessitates creativity. The essence lies in utilizing the space for high-intensity bodyweight workouts that require minimal room. Bodyweight exercises are not only convenient and cost-effective, they are also remarkably versatile. Here's what to keep in mind:

- **Space Optimization**: Every inch counts. You'll use walls, the edge of the tub, and even the sink strategically.

- **Safety First**: Ensure non-slip mats are in place and the floor is dry to prevent injuries.

- **Multi-functional Movements**: Select exercises that target multiple muscle groups at once.

- **Time Efficiency**: Workouts should be short bursts, aligning with high-intensity interval training (HIIT) principles.

- **Routine Variability**: Rotate exercises to target different muscle groups and avoid monotony.

Practical Implementation

Transform your bathroom into a mini-gym with these actionable steps:

1. **Warm-Up**: Begin with high knees or jog in place to get your heart rate up.

2. **Decline Push-Ups**: Place your feet on the edge of the tub, hands on the floor for an intense push-up variation.

3. **Tricep Dips**: Use the side of the tub or a sturdy sink to perform tricep dips.

4. **Wall Sit**: Lean against the wall with legs at a 90-degree angle, as if sitting on a chair.

5. **Step-Ups**: Utilize the side of the tub as a stepper for leg work.

6. **Towel Rows**: For back exercises, hold the ends of a towel, place feet against the base of the door and lean back, then row.

7. **Bathroom Squats**: Stand in front of the toilet, lower into a squat as if sitting down, and stand back up.

8. **Calf Raises**: Stand on the edge of a raised surface, like a sturdy bathmat, and rise onto your toes, then lower.

9. **Incline Push-Ups**: Place hands on the edge of the sink for a less intense push-up variation.

Consistency and Evaluation

Adhering to a routine is crucial for seeing results. Monitor your progress with a simple tracking system. Evaluate your performance on a weekly basis. Adjust the difficulty by increasing repetitions or holding positions for a longer duration as your strength improves.

- **Weekly Check-in**: Look back at your workouts, reflect on achievements and areas needing improvement.

- **Exercise Log**: Keep a record of reps, sets, and hold times to track progress.

- **Rest Days**: Incorporate rest into your routine to allow muscles to recover.

Remember, your bathroom can be the unexpected ally in your fitness quest, harnessing the power of bodyweight training in a space no larger than a closet. Dedication and creativity are your ticket to making the most of every square inch.

PARK BENCH WORKOUT: TONE UP IN THE OUTDOORS

The Key Ideas

Accessibility: Park benches are ubiquitous and can be the foundation of an effective workout routine. Enjoying the outdoors while exercising can boost your mood and provide a change of scenery from the gym.

Versatility: A variety of exercises targeting different muscle groups can be performed using just a park bench. This can offer a full-body workout without any additional equipment.

Adaptability: Park bench workouts can be modified to suit different fitness levels. Add repetitions or sets, increase the speed of execution, or include additional elements like jumps or weights as you progress.

Functionality: The exercises mimic natural movements and daily activities, promoting functional fitness that benefits your everyday life.

Practical Implementation

1. **Bench Push-Ups:**

   - Hands on the bench, feet on the ground.

- Lower your body, keeping your back straight.

   - Press back up to the starting position.

2. **Bench Dips:**

   - Sit on the bench with hands next to hips.

   - Slide off with your legs extended.

   - Bend and extend your arms to dip down and up.

3. **Step-Ups:**

   - Face the bench and step up with one foot.

   - Follow with the other, then step down and repeat.

4. **Bench Squats:**

   - Stand with your back to the bench.

   - Lower until you lightly touch the seat, then return to standing.

5. **Plank with Feet Elevated:**

   - Place your forearms on the ground and feet on the bench.

   - Hold a straight line from shoulders to heels.

6. **Bench Lunges:**

   - Place one foot on the bench behind you.

   - Lower into a lunge, then push back up.

7. **Incline Mountain Climbers:**

   - Hands on the bench, in a push-up position.

   - Alternately draw knees to chest at a brisk pace.

8. **Bench Side Planks:**

   ○ Place one forearm on the bench, stack your feet or place one in front of the other.

   ○ Lift hips to make a straight line with your body.

9. **Leg Swings:**

   ○ Hold onto the back of the bench for support.

   ○ Swing one leg forward and backward, then side to side before switching legs.

10. **Bench Pike Press:**

   ○ Hands on a bench, hips high in a pike position.

   ○ Bend your arms to lower your head towards the bench, then push back up.

Warm-Up and Cooldown:

- Spend 5 minutes walking or jogging around the park.

- Stretch major muscle groups post-workout.

Consistency and Evaluation

Commitment: Aim for 3–4 park bench sessions per week. Consistency is key to seeing results.

Progress Tracking: Keep a log of your repetitions, sets, and any added difficulty. This will help you measure your progress and motivate you toward your goals.

Listen to Your Body: Pay attention to your form and any signs of strain. Adjust the workout as necessary to avoid injury.

Seek Challenge and Variety: Incrementally increase the intensity as you become stronger. This might mean adding jumps to step-ups or increasing the speed and duration of your workout.

Reflect and Reward: Acknowledge your achievements, no matter how small, and treat yourself to rest days to recover. Fitness is a journey, and every step counts toward your overall well-being.

KETTLEBELL KOMBAT: 9-MINUTE BLAST

The Key Ideas

- **Efficiency and Effectiveness**: Combining cardiovascular and strength training, kettlebell exercises maximize calorie-burn and muscle engagement in minimal time.

- **Full-Body Workout**: Engage multiple muscle groups simultaneously for comprehensive fitness.

- **Variety of Movements**: Utilize dynamic kettlebell moves that mimic real-world activities and combat movements for improved functional strength.

- **Progressive Overload**: Gradually increase weight or intensity to challenge your body and prevent plateaus.

- **Mind-Muscle Connection**: Stay mentally engaged to ensure proper form, maximizing benefits and reducing the risk of injury.

Practical Implementation

1. **Selecting Your Kettlebell**:

    ◦ Start with a weight that challenges you but allows you to maintain proper form. For most beginners, 8-16 kg is appropriate depending on fitness level and gender.

2. **Warm-Up (1 minute)**:

    ◦ Begin with dynamic stretches focusing on shoulders, hips, and hamstrings.

3. **The Kettlebell Kombat Circuit**: Perform each exercise for 45 seconds with a 15-second rest in between. Complete two rounds.

4. **Swing**: The foundational kettlebell movement for power and explosiveness.

    ◦ **Goblet Squat**: Engages the core, quads, and glutes.

    ◦ **One-Arm Row**: Builds back strength and challenges core stability.

    ◦ **Hardstyle Plank**: An intense core stabilizer.

    ◦ **Boxers' Snatch**: Mimics a punching movement, combining cardiovascular with power training.

    ◦ **Windmill**: Increases shoulder stability and targets obliques.

5. **Cooldown (1 minute)**:

    ◦ End with static stretching, focusing on the muscles worked.

Consistency and Evaluation

- **Measure Progress**: Track the weight of your kettlebell, repetitions per set, and overall workout intensity. Over time, all should increase.

- **Listen to Your Body**: Rest when required, and step back if form is compromised.

Key Points for Evaluation:

- **Strength Gains**: Are you able to increase the kettlebell weight over time?

- **Endurance Improvement**: Can you perform more reps or require shorter rest periods?

- **Posture and Form**: Is your kettlebell technique improving?

- **Physical Feedback**: Reduced fatigue and improved ease in daily activities indicate functional fitness gains.

Consistent application and mindful execution will deliver significant improvements in fitness even with just 9 minutes.

COMMUTE CYCLE: INTERVAL TRAINING ON YOUR RIDE HOME

The Key Ideas

Turn your homeward cycle into a productive exercise. The concept is simple: intersperse bouts of high-intensity pedaling with intervals of easy riding. This approach, known as High-Intensity Interval Training (HIIT), can dramatically improve your cardiovascular health and burn calories efficiently.

• **Intensity Over Duration**: Short, intense bursts followed by recovery periods.

• **Adaptability**: Works for any distance and does not require additional time.

• **Accessibility**: No special equipment needed, beyond a bike.

Practical Implementation

1. **Start with a Warm-up**: Begin with 5-10 minutes of steady, moderate-paced cycling to prepare your body.

2. **Intervals**: After warming up:

   ○ Sprint for 30 seconds at maximum effort.

- Cycle casually for 2 minutes. This is your recovery phase.

- Repeat this cycle for the duration of your commute.

3. **Cool Down**: End your ride with a 5-minute easy pace to aid in recovery.

4. **Track Your Progress**:

- Use a simple cycle computer or smartphone app to track times and monitor improvement.

5. **Safety First**:

- Wear appropriate gear, including a helmet and visible clothing.

- Choose safe routes and ensure your bike is well-maintained.

Tips for Success:

- Prioritize seated sprints to build endurance.

- Stand up periodically to engage different muscle groups.

- Alternate your route to include hills for natural resistance training.

Consistency and Evaluation

- **Set a Schedule**: Aim to perform interval training 2-3 times a week.

- **Measure Improvement**: Every two weeks, evaluate your fitness gains:

- Can you sprint longer?

- Has your recovery time decreased?

- Are you feeling stronger on the bike?

- **Listen to Your Body**:

  - Adjust intervals and intensity based on physical condition.

  - Take note of any pain or discomfort. Rest if needed.

Final Thought: Interval training can transform a mundane commute into a dynamic workout. With no extra time spent, you can enhance your fitness, boost your energy levels, and enjoy an energizing ride home.

FAST TRACK TO FLEXIBILITY: QUICK STRETCH TECHNIQUES

The Key Ideas

Flexibility is both a component of fitness and a facet of overall well-being. Gaining it doesn't require extensive hours; it can fit into your bustling life. Here's how:

• **Dynamic Stretching:** Rapid, controlled leg and arm swings that take you (gently!) to the limits of your range of motion.

• **Static Stretching After Exercise:** Holding a stretch for 20-30 seconds, ideally post-workout when muscles are warm.

• **PNF Stretching:** Proprioceptive Neuromuscular Facilitation involves contracting and stretching the target muscle group.

• **Short, Daily Sessions:** Even 5-10 minutes a day can make a remarkable difference.

Practical Implementation

To incorporate these ideas into your everyday life, follow these guidelines:

1. **Warm-Up with Dynamic Stretches:** Start with 5 minutes of light cardio, then move on to gentle swings of your arms and legs. Examples include:

   - Leg swings, side-to-side and front-to-back

   - Arm circles, small to large

   - Hip circles and twists

2. **Incorporate Stretching Post-Exercise:** Directly after your workout, focus on static stretches such as:

   - Touching your toes for hamstring and back flexibility

   - Quadricep stretch by pulling your foot to your buttock

   - Calf stretch against a wall or curb

3. **Try PNF Stretching Once a Week:** Use caution as these are advanced:

   - Hold a stretch, then contract the muscle for 5 seconds, release, and stretch further.

4. **Yoga or Pilates Classes:** Both practices incorporate strength and flexibility work that can complement your stretching routine.

5. **Stay Motivated with Variety:** Vary your stretches to keep your routine engaging. Different styles like yoga, tai chi, or dance can offer new types of flexibility training.

Consistency and Evaluation

Consistency is your golden ticket. To evaluate and maintain progress:

- **Track Your Progress:** Note your starting flexibility level and monitor changes weekly.

- **Set Realistic Goals:** Focus on attainable improvements to motivate continued effort.

- **Listen to Your Body:** Push for progress but never force a stretch to the point of pain.

Maintaining a flexible body requires regular attention but doesn't have to dominate your schedule. By weaving these techniques into your routine, incremental improvements will accumulate, leading to significant gains in flexibility.

SUPERMARKET SHAPE-UP: INCORPORATING FITNESS INTO ERRANDS

The Key Ideas

Regular trips to the supermarket can double as opportunities for physical activity. Here are the core concepts:

- **Leveraging Time**: Utilize the time spent shopping to include exercise, making the most of every minute.

- **Incorporating Movement**: Integrate simple exercises that can be done while moving through the aisles.

- **Making it Fun**: Approach fitness during errands as a playful addition to routine, not a chore.

- **Safety First**: Ensure that exercises don't obstruct aisles or create hazards for other shoppers.

Practical Implementation

Begin with these steps to blend fitness into your shopping routine:

1. **Warm-Up**: Start with a brisk five-minute walk around the parking lot before entering the store.

2. **Grocery Lunges**: Perform lunges while pushing the cart down the aisle.

3. **Shelf Reaches**: Use high and low shelf items to stretch and strengthen arms and legs.

4. **Calf Raises**: While standing in line, rise onto your toes and back down to work your calf muscles.

5. **Squat and Lift**: Safely incorporate squats when lifting heavier items into your cart.

6. **Tighten Core**: Engage your abdominal muscles as you walk around the store.

7. **Cool Down**: Finish with a five-minute walk around the store or parking lot at a slower pace to cool down.

Remember, select exercises suitable for your fitness level and mindful of the space and people around you.

Consistency and Evaluation

To see results:

• **Schedule Regularity**: Aim to shop on a set schedule to create a consistent workout routine.

• **Track Progress**: Consider using a fitness tracker to monitor steps taken and calories burned.

• **Listen to Your Body**: Pay attention to how your body feels during and after the workout.

• **Adjust as Needed**: Modify the intensity and variety of exercises based on comfort and progression.

In conclusion, supermarket trips are an untapped resource for incorporating exercise into your day. By following these straightforward strategies, you can enhance your health while completing necessary errands.

QUICK FOOTWORK: AGILITY LADDER DRILLS IN 5 MINUTES

The Key Ideas

Speed and agility are critical components in many sports and everyday activities. Agility ladder drills are designed to enhance these attributes by improving foot speed, coordination, and spatial awareness. Here's the core of what you need to know:

• **Purpose of Agility Ladder Drills**: Enhance your footwork, boost coordination, and increase cardiovascular fitness in a short time frame.

• **Intensity**: Aim for high intensity to capitalize on the workout's brief duration.

• **Focus**: Quality over quantity. Concentrate on the precision of movement rather than speed, especially when learning new patterns.

Practical Implementation

Start with a quick warm-up, such as jogging or jumping jacks, to prepare your muscles and increase heart rate. Here's how to execute a 5-minute ladder drill session:

1. **Forward Zig-Zag Run**:

   - Start at one end of the ladder.

   - Run through the ladder, placing one foot in each square.

   - Keep your knees up and maintain a forward lean.

2. **Lateral High Knees**:

   - Face sideways, leading with your right side.

   - Lift knees high and step into each box rapidly.

   - Reach the end, switch to lead with your left side, and repeat.

3. **In-and-Out Hop Scotch**:

   - Jump with both feet into the first square.

   - Hop into a split stance with one foot inside the ladder and the other outside.

   - Continue alternating the in-and-out pattern down the ladder.

4. **Ickey Shuffle**:

   - Start with your right foot in the first square.

   - Step in with the left foot, and then step out with the right foot to the side.

   - Progress down the ladder by repeating the three-step pattern.

5. **Two-Footed Bunny Hops**:

    ○ Begin at one end with feet shoulder-width apart.

    ○ Hop forward, landing in each square on both feet simultaneously.

    ○ Keep your movements compact and springs quick.

Use a timer and perform each drill for 45 seconds, followed by 15 seconds of rest, to round out your 5-minute session.

Consistency and Evaluation

To reap the benefits of agility ladder drills, integrate them into your routine at least three times a week. Assess your progress by:

• **Timing Drills**: Record the time it takes to complete a drill without errors. Look for improvements in speed as you progress.

• **Footwork Accuracy**: Monitor the precision of your steps. Less fumbling translates to better coordination.

• **Cardiovascular Endurance**: Notice if you're less winded after a complete session over time.

In conclusion, these agile ladder drills pack a punch in a compact five minutes. Make them a staple for a nimble, well-coordinated, and faster you.

DYNAMIC DUO: PARTNER WORKOUTS FOR THE TIME-STARVED

The Key Ideas

Partner workouts are an effective strategy for those struggling to find time for fitness. They incorporate social interaction, motivation, and accountability, making exercise more enjoyable and efficient.

- **Mutual Motivation**: Your workout partner pushes you, ensuring you both get the most from each session.

- **Shared Time**: Combining social time with exercise, partner workouts kill two birds with one stone.

- **Diverse Activities**: Workouts can range from traditional exercises to sports or active games.

- **Space Efficiency**: Many partner exercises require minimal equipment or space.

- **Adaptability**: Suits varying fitness levels and can be tailored to individual goals.

Practical Implementation

Start with a clear plan and choose exercises that keep you both engaged and challenged. Here is a step-by-step guide:

1. **Select a Compatible Partner**: Find someone with similar fitness goals and availability.

2. **Set Common Goals**: Agree on what you both want to achieve and set a timeline.

3. **Plan Your Workouts**: Choose exercises that are conducive to partnership, like medicine ball tosses, partner planks, or back-to-back squats.

4. **Equip Minimally**: Use bodyweight movements or portable equipment like resistance bands.

5. **Synchronize Schedules**: Commit to regular sessions, whether that's early mornings, lunch breaks, or evenings.

Sample Workout Routine

- **Warm-up** (5 minutes): Joint mobility exercises and light cardio.

- **Main Set** (20 minutes):

  - Circuit of bodyweight exercises: Push-ups, sit-ups, partner-assisted squats, and back-to-back wall sits.

  - Cardio boost: Partner tag, shadow boxing, or jump rope.

- **Cool Down** (5 minutes): Stretching and relaxation exercises.

Consistency and Evaluation

Consistent practice and regular assessments are key to success.

- **Track Progress**: Use a shared log to monitor workouts and improvements.

- **Feedback Loop**: Offer constructive criticism and celebrate successes together.

- **Adjust Regularly**: Modify the routine as you both progress to maintain challenge and interest.

- **Stay Accountable**: Check in with each other to maintain a steady routine.

In conclusion, partner workouts are a time-efficient means to integrate fitness into a busy life. They foster a sense of camaraderie and shared purpose, making the commitment to exercise a collective endeavor.

5-MINUTE MEDITATION & MINDFULNESS FOR RECOVERY

The Key Ideas

Meditation and mindfulness are not just buzzwords; they are valuable tools for recovery and rejuvenation. Engaging in a 5-minute meditation session can reset your stress levels, improve focus, and support overall well-being. These practices encourage a moment-to-moment awareness of our thoughts, feelings, bodily sensations, and surrounding environment.

- **Brief and Consistent**: Short, daily practices can be more beneficial than occasional, longer sessions.

- **Accessible**: No special equipment or environments are required—practice anywhere, anytime.

- **Adaptive**: Can be tailored to fit your personal recovery needs, whether physical, emotional, or mental.

Practical Implementation

Starting Your Practice

- **Find a Quiet Space**: Minimize distractions. A calm environment aids focus.

- **Comfortable Position**: Sit or lie in a comfortable position. Keep your back straight to promote alertness.

- **Set a Timer**: Use a timer for five minutes to help you fully engage without clock-watching.

Techniques

1. **Deep Breathing**:

   - Focus on slow, deep breaths.

   - Inhale through the nose, expanding your belly, then chest.

   - Exhale through the mouth, releasing all tension.

2. **Body Scan**:

   - Start at your toes and move upwards.

   - Notice each body part without judgment; release tension as you go.

3. **Mantra Repetition**:

   - Choose a word or phrase that resonates with your recovery.

   - Silently repeat it, letting it anchor your thoughts.

4. **Mindful Observation**:

   - Pick an object within your view.

   - Note its shape, color, texture, and other traits without evaluation.

During Meditation

- **Acknowledge Distractions**: Gently bring your focus back without criticism.

- **Allow Thoughts to Pass**: Visualize them as clouds drifting by.

- **Stay Present**: If you drift, return to your breath or chosen focal point.

Consistency and Evaluation

Building a Routine

- **Same Time Daily**: A regular schedule promotes habit formation.

- **Post-Workout**: Incorporate meditation into your cool-down routine.

- **Post-Stress**: After high stress, use meditation as a recovery tool.

Assessing Progress

- **Mood Tracking**: Keep a journal to observe mood changes over time.

- **Physical Recovery**: Note reductions in muscle tension or stress-related symptoms.

- **Cognitive Clarity**: Are you experiencing increased focus or creativity post-meditation?

Through consistent practice and evaluation, 5-minute meditation and mindfulness can become a transformative aspect of your recovery regimen. Remember, the goal is not perfection, but rather presence and progress.

TV TIME TONING: EXERCISE DURING COMMERCIALS

The Key Ideas

Turn idle minutes into a fitness opportunity. Maximize commercial breaks during TV time as exercise segments. This approach can seamlessly integrate physical activity into your daily routine without overwhelming your schedule. Here are the essential concepts to understand:

- **Micro Workout Philosophy**: Short bursts of exercise can compound into significant health benefits.

- **Accessibility**: Your living room becomes your gym, no special equipment needed.

- **Flexibility**: Choose exercises based on your current fitness level and interests.

- **Commitment-Free**: This method allows for commitment on a per-commercial basis, resolving the issue of finding 'big blocks' of time for exercise.

Practical Implementation

Start using commercial breaks as a cue for activity. Follow this step-by-step process:

1. **Prepare Your Space**: Clear a small workout area in front of your TV.

2. **Create a Routine List**: Have a list of exercises ready for variety and to prevent decision fatigue. Include bodyweight exercises like push-ups, sit-ups, squats, lunges, or jumping jacks.

3. **Warm-Up**: Initiate with light stretching during the show to prevent injury.

4. **Sequence Your Workouts**: Alternate between upper body, lower body, and core exercises.

5. **Use Commercial Length as a Timer**: A standard commercial break lasts about 2-3 minutes, perfect for sets or intervals.

6. **Cool Down**: Use the final commercial break for slower exercises and stretching.

Mimic the structure:

- **First Break**: Lower body – lunges and squats

- **Second Break**: Core – planks and sit-ups

- **Third Break**: Upper body – push-ups and arm circles

- **Fourth Break**: Flexibility – stretching and yoga poses

Consistency and Evaluation

To achieve tangible results, consistency is crucial. Track your progress:

- **Log Your Activity**: Jot down each set of exercises performed during commercials.

- **Measure Frequency**: Aim to exercise during commercials at least five days a week.

- **Assess Intensity**: Gradually increase repetitions or extend the duration for each exercise.

Evaluate your fitness improvements monthly. Look for changes in your endurance, strength, and flexibility. Adjust your routine as you advance, challenging yourself with new or modified exercises. Celebrate small victories and stay flexible with your routine to maintain your motivation. Remember, this is about making the most of your time, not over-exerting yourself. Be cautious, listen to your body, and enjoy the compounded benefits of these mini workouts.

SWIFT SWISS BALL SCULPTING SESSION

The Key Ideas

Swiss balls, also known as stability balls, are dynamic tools for developing balance, muscle tone, and core strength. The unique benefits of this exercise apparatus derive from its instability, which forces the recruitment of numerous muscles to maintain balance. Here are the key ideas you need to consider before starting:

- **Muscle Engagement:** Training with a Swiss ball involves multiple muscle groups, especially the core, enhancing overall stability and posture.

- **Balance and Coordination:** Using an unstable surface increases proprioception, making your body more aware of its positioning in space.

- **Adjusted Intensity:** You can easily scale the difficulty of exercises up or down by modifying your body position or the ball's placement.

Practical Implementation

To effectively incorporate the Swiss ball into your training, follow these guidelines:

1. **Select the Right Size Ball**: Your knees should be at a right angle when sitting on the ball with feet flat on the floor.

2. **Warm-Up**: Start with a 5-minute dynamic stretching routine to prepare your muscles.

3. **The Exercises**:

   ○ *Swiss Ball Planks*: Strengthens the core. Forearms on the ball, legs extended, hold a straight line from head to heels.

   ○ *Ball Wall Squats*: Targets glutes and quads. Place ball between your lower back and the wall while performing squats.

   ○ *Hamstring Curls*: Lying on your back, feet on the ball, lift your hips and roll the ball towards you.

   ○ *Ball Push-Ups*: For the chest and core. Feet on the ball, perform a push-up with hands on the ground.

   ○ *Jackknife*: Targets abdominals. With shins on the ball and hands on the floor, tuck your knees towards your chest.

4. **Duration and Repetitions**: Start with 10-15 reps per exercise. Aim for two sets initially, increasing as you improve.

5. **Cool Down**: Conclude your session with 5-10 minutes of static stretching for muscle recovery.

Consistency and Evaluation

To truly reap the benefits of your Swiss ball workouts, integrate these sessions into your fitness plan 2-3 times weekly. Monitor your progress by noting increases in reps or sets, as well as improvements in form and control.

• **Track Consistency**: Maintain a workout log.

• **Self-evaluate Form**: Use a mirror or record yourself to check technique.

• **Listen to Your Body**: Adjust intensity based on your comfort and challenge levels.

Remember, to sculpt your body effectively, patience and perseverance are as important as the exercises themselves. Stay committed, and you will see the transformation.

SPEEDY KICKBOXING BASICS: HIT AND HUSTLE

The Key Ideas

Lesson 1: Understand the Fundamentals Kickboxing combines martial arts techniques with fast-paced cardio. Learning the basics —stances, punches, kicks, and movements—is essential.

Lesson 2: Efficient Workout Design Focus on interval training. Combine high-intensity bursts with brief periods of rest. This maximizes calorie burn and hones technique in shorter sessions.

Lesson 3: Technique Over Power Initially, prioritize form over force. Proper technique ensures maximum efficiency and minimizes injury.

Practical Implementation

1. Warm-Up (5 minutes)

- **Jog in place**: Elevate your heart rate.

- **Arm circles and leg raises**: Loosen joints and increase mobility.

2. Fundamental Stances and Movements (5 minutes)

- **Boxer's shuffle**: Stay light on your feet.
- **Guard position**: Hands up to protect the face.

3. Techniques (10 minutes)

- **Jab**: Quick, straight punch from the lead hand.
- **Cross**: Powerful punch from the back hand.
- **Hook**: Rounded punch aimed at the side of your opponent's head/body.
- **Uppercut**: Upward punch from the waist, targeting the chin.
- **Front Kick**: Snap kick from the lead leg.
- **Roundhouse Kick**: Powerful kick executing a circular motion.

4. Drills and Combinations (10 minutes)

- Craft a series of 3-4 move combos, repeating for 2-3 minutes, then switch.
- Example: Jab, cross, hook, and a front kick.

5. Interval Training (10 minutes)

- **20 seconds**: Intense bursts of a combo-set.
- **10 seconds**: Rest or active recovery like light jogging.

6. Cool Down (5 minutes)

- **Shadowboxing**: Low intensity to lower the heart rate.
- **Stretching**: Focus on flexibility to aid recovery.

Consistency and Evaluation

Consistency Practice regularly, aiming for at least 3 times a week. Equal focus on all techniques ensures structured progress.

Evaluation After four weeks, assess improvements in:

- Speed and power of strikes.

- Cardiovascular endurance.

- Overall technique fluency.

Monitor each session's intensity and adjust to steadily increase your threshold. This feedback will guide you to refine your workouts for continuous improvement.

POWER PLANKING VARIATIONS: BEYOND THE BASICS

The Key Ideas

Planking, a core-strengthening exercise, is a staple in fitness routines. Traditional planks lay the foundation for a strong, stable midsection. However, to maximize gains and prevent plateaus, introducing variations is essential.

Progressive Overload

- Incremental increases in intensity keep muscles adapting.

- Variations add complexity and resistance, promoting continuous improvement.

Engaging Multiple Muscle Groups

- Variations engage secondary muscles, offering a more comprehensive workout.

- Balancing and dynamic movements enlist stabilizing muscles.

Preventing Boredom and Plateaus

- Diverse exercises maintain motivation.

• Switching routines challenges the body in new ways, averting performance stagnation.

Practical Implementation

To evolve your standard plank routine, incorporate the following variations:

1. **Side Planks**

   ○ Targets obliques, enhances lateral stability.

   ○ Keep body in a straight line from head to feet, lifting hips high.

2. **Plank with Leg Lift**

   ○ Strengthens glutes and lower back.

   ○ Alternate lifting each leg, maintaining a solid core.

3. **Plank with Arm Lift**

   ○ Engages upper back, shoulders, and core.

   ○ Extend one arm at a time, keeping the body level.

4. **Spiderman Plank**

   ○ Activates obliques, chest, and hip flexors.

   ○ Bring each knee to the corresponding elbow, alternating sides.

5. **Plank Jacks**

   ○ Incorporates cardio, targets inner and outer thighs.

   ○ Jump feet in and out like a jumping jack while maintaining plank form.

6. **Mountain Climbers**

   ○ Elevates heart rate, fosters agility and core strength.

   ○ Drive knees towards the chest in rapid succession.

7. **Plank Ups**

   ○ Builds upper body strength and core stability.

   ○ Alternate between forearm plank and push-up position.

8. **Reverse Plank**

   ○ Emphasizes lower back, glutes, and hamstrings.

   ○ Sit on the floor, legs extended, elevate body on hands or elbows.

Use a mix of these variations within a workout or across a training week to ensure a comprehensive core challenge.

Consistency and Evaluation

Schedule Regularity

- Set a routine that integrates plank variations 3-4 times a week.

- Aim for 2-3 sets of each variation, holding or performing repetitions for 20-60 seconds.

Progress Tracking

- Monitor hold times and repetitions – improvements indicate enhanced core strength.

- Use a workout diary or app for accountability.

Technique Check-Ins

- Prioritize form over duration or intensity to prevent injury.

- Periodically reassess technique, especially when fatigue sets in.

Listen to Your Body

- Quality is paramount; avoid pushing through pain.

- Adjust variations to accommodate any injuries or strain.

By integrating these power planking variations into your regimen, you expand and refine your core strength, ensuring your quick workouts remain effective and engaging. Adopt these practices for a resilient and dynamic core, and reap the benefits of advanced fitness within a time-compressed schedule.

ZEN IN TEN: SPEEDY TAI CHI STRETCH

The Key Ideas

Tai Chi, an ancient Chinese martial art, promotes harmony and relaxation. Its core revolves around flowing movements and deep breathing. The purpose of this chapter is to distill its essence into a 10-minute routine that anyone can incorporate into a busy schedule. With just 10 minutes, this modified Tai Chi sequence aims to reduce stress, improve your flexibility, and enhance mental clarity.

Practical Implementation

Morning Awakening (2 minutes)

- Stand with feet shoulder-width apart.

- Gently raise your arms to the sides and above your head as you inhale deeply.

- Exhale slowly, lowering your arms back down.

- Repeat this flowing motion, synchronizing it with your breath.

Windmill Hand Sways (1 minute)

- Raise one arm up beside your head while simultaneously lowering the other.

- Bend your torso slightly as if swaying in the wind.

- Inhale as your hand goes up, exhale as it goes down.

- Alternate smoothly to create a rhythm.

Wrist Circles (1 minute)

- Extend your arms outward, parallel to the ground.

- Rotate your wrists gently, first clockwise, then counter-clockwise.

- Focus on releasing tension with each rotation.

The Expanding Sphere(2 minutes)

- Interlace your fingers with palms facing outward.

- As you inhale, expand your arms in front of you, imagining you are holding a large sphere.

- Exhale and draw the sphere close, bringing your elbows towards your body.

- Maintain fluid motions, breathing deeply.

The Majestic Crane (2 minutes)

- From a standing position, slowly shift your weight onto one leg.

- Simultaneously lift the opposite knee and balance briefly.

- Arms mimic the wings of a crane as you maintain balance.

- Alternate legs, moving gracefully.

Embracing the Tree (2 minutes)

- Stand with knees slightly bent, feet shoulder-width apart.
- Hold arms rounded in front of you as if embracing a large tree.
- Hold the position, breathe deeply.
- Imagine drawing energy from the tree with each breath.

Closing Reflection (1 minute)

- Stand quietly, hands by your sides.
- Take deep, even breaths.
- Reflect on the sensation of calm and stretch in your body.

Consistency and Evaluation

Consistency is key to feeling the benefits of Tai Chi, even with just 10 minutes a day. Assess your stress levels before and after the stretch. Notice any changes: are your muscles more relaxed? Do you feel more grounded and centered? Track these subtle shifts daily to truly tap into Tai Chi's transformative power.

RESTROOM REFRESHERS: SWIFT WORKOUTS FOR ROAD WARRIORS

The Key Ideas

Staying active on the road can be a significant challenge. Unexpected delays, cramped seating, and limited space needn't bar you from keeping fit. Restroom refreshers are a series of quick, efficient exercises designed to be done in small spaces, making them perfect for travelers.

- **Utility Over Space:** Leveraging the small space of a restroom or similarly confined area for a full-body workout.

- **Privacy:** Restrooms offer privacy for exercises that may feel awkward in public spaces.

- **Time-Efficiency:** Focusing on exercises that give you the most benefits in a short period.

- **Adaptability:** Using body weight for resistance and adapting exercises to match fitness levels.

Practical Implementation

To implement these swift workouts, follow these steps:

1. Warm-Up: Start by doing a quick set of jumping jacks or running in place to get the blood flowing.

2. Leg Work: Move into air squats or wall sits for a lower body burn.

3. Upper Body: Use countertop push-ups (against the sink area) to build upper body strength.

4. Core Focus: Perform standing oblique crunches or toe touches for core conditioning.

5. Cool Down: End with stretching exercises to reduce soreness and aid recovery.

Example Routine:

- **20 sec** of running in place
- **15 air squats**
- **10 countertop push-ups**
- **20 sec** of standing oblique crunches (10 sec per side)
- **1 minute** stretching (neck, arm, calf stretches, and deep breathing)

Adjust the number of repetitions and sets based on your time availability and fitness level.

Consistency and Evaluation

Consistency is crucial. Aim to incorporate these workouts into your daily routine, regardless of where you are. Evaluate your progress by noting any improvements in your capacity to perform the exercises or increases in the number of repetitions over time.

- **Daily Goals:** Set a goal to perform this workout at least once a day.

- **Record Keeping:** Keep a log of your workouts in a journal or a mobile app.

- **Adaptation:** As you get stronger, increase the difficulty by adding more repetitions or sets.

- **Listen to Your Body:** If an exercise feels wrong, modify it to suit your needs.

Remember, the objective is not perfection but consistent effort over time.

TARGETED GLUTES & LEGS: QUICK LOWER BODY BURNER

The Key Ideas

When time is scarce, and you aim to strengthen and tone your lower body effectively, targeted workouts for glutes and legs can make a meaningful impact. Through compound exercises that recruit multiple muscle groups, you can achieve a noteworthy burn in a brief period.

- **Efficiency in Movements**: Select exercises that engage a wide range of muscles simultaneously, maximizing calorie burn.

- **Intensity**: Integrate high-intensity intervals to increase the heart rate and optimize fat loss.

- **Progressive Overload**: Gradually increase the difficulty of exercises to continue challenging your muscles.

- **Mind-Muscle Connection**: Focus on the muscle being targeted to improve contraction and effectiveness.

Practical Implementation

To put these concepts into action, a concise, potent routine is key. This plan can be executed in under 20 minutes and requires minimal equipment.

1. **Warm-Up** (3 minutes):

   ○ Light jogging or jumping jacks

   ○ Dynamic stretches: leg swings, hip circles

2. **Workout Routine**:

Do each exercise for 45 seconds followed by 15 seconds rest. Complete the circuit twice.

- Squats: Stand with feet shoulder-width apart, lower into a squat, keep chest up.

  ○ Lunges: Alternate legs stepping forward into a lunge, maintain upright posture.

  ○ Glute Bridges: Lie on your back, feet planted, lift hips by squeezing glutes.

  ○ Deadlifts: With dumbbells, hinge at hips, keep back straight, lift to standing.

  ○ Lateral Leg Raises: Lying on your side, lift the upper leg, pause, then lower.

- **Cool Down** (3 minutes):

  ○ Static stretches: hamstring stretch, quad stretch, glute stretch

Consistency and Evaluation

Consistency is the linchpin of success in any fitness regimen. Aiming to perform this routine 3 times a week can yield marked improvements in strength and muscle tone. It can be scaled up or down according to your fitness level.

Evaluation: Keep a workout journal. Note improvements in:

- Repetitions and sets over time

- The ease of performing exercises

- Visual changes in muscle tone

- Upgrades in weights or resistance

Regular assessments every three to four weeks can help you stay on track and adjust your routine for continued progress.

FAST AND FURIOUS: SPEED ENDURANCE DRILLS

The Key Ideas

Speed endurance is the ability to maintain high-speed running or work output at near-maximum pace for as long as possible. It's critical for athletes in sports like soccer, basketball, and track and field, but it's just as beneficial for the everyday fitness enthusiast seeking efficiency and effectiveness from their workouts.

The core principles of developing speed endurance are:

- **Intensity**: Workouts must be high effort.

- **Rest**: Adequate recovery is necessary to repeat efforts at high intensity.

- **Progression**: Gradually increasing the difficulty of drills over time.

Practical Implementation

1. **Dynamic Warm-Up**: Kickstart each session with 5-10 minutes of dynamic stretches to prepare your muscles and cardiovascular system—think high knees, leg swings, and arm circles.

2. **Interval Training**:

   ◦ Run hard for a set distance or time (e.g., 100 meters or 45 seconds).

   ◦ Follow with a recovery period of walking or slow jogging for double the time or distance.

   ◦ Repeat for 6 to 12 cycles depending on your fitness level.

3. **Hill Workouts**:

   ◦ Find a moderate hill. Sprint up for 30 seconds at max effort.

   ◦ Walk back down at a leisurely pace for recovery.

   ◦ Perform 6 to 10 repetitions.

4. **Fartlek Training**:

   ◦ During a steady-state run, inject periods of 30-60 seconds of sprinting.

   ◦ Follow each burst with 1-2 minutes of jogging or walking to recover.

   ◦ Continue this pattern for 20-30 minutes.

5. **Tempo Runs**:

   ◦ Run for a set distance or time (e.g., 3 miles or 20 minutes) at a challenging but sustainable pace.

   ◦ Push the pace just outside your comfort zone.

6. **Plyometric Drills**:

   ◦ Include exercises like jump squats, box jumps, and burpees.

   ◦ Perform 3 sets of 8-12 reps with proper form.

7. **Speed Ladders and Agility Drills:**

   ◦ Fast feet through agility ladders improve quickness and footwork.

   ◦ Drills should be short in duration (20-30 seconds) and high in intensity.

Consistency and Evaluation

To reap benefits:

- Aim to include speed endurance drills 2-3 times per week.

- Record times, distances, and the intensity of each drill to track improvement.

- Listen to your body and ensure you're getting enough rest.

Always incorporate 48-72 hours of recovery time between intense speed workouts to allow for adaptation and growth.

Remember: Overtraining can lead to injury and setbacks. Keep a balanced approach for sustainable progress. Be patient; speed endurance doesn't develop overnight but with consistent effort, improvements will come.

NO-EQUIPMENT NEEDED: 9-MINUTE NINJA MOVES

The Key Ideas

You have nine minutes and your body: that's all you need. These dynamic, ninja-inspired moves are designed to improve agility, strength, and cardiovascular health. They tap into bodyweight training, demanding multi-directional movement, speed, and precision. The key is intensity; push hard for short bursts and maximize the efficiency of a short workout.

- **Total Body Engagement**: Each move targets multiple muscle groups simultaneously.

- **High Intensity**: Quick, explosive actions increase heart rate.

- **Agility and Coordination**: Fast-paced transitions require and build coordination.

- **Space-Efficient**: Small workout area needed.

- **Time-Efficient**: Complete workout within nine minutes.

Practical Implementation

Begin with a quick warm-up to prepare your body for intense movement. Then, cycle through these three ninja moves, aiming for three sets, which fits neatly into nine minutes.

1. **Shinobi Shuffle**: (30 seconds)

   - Stand with feet shoulder-width apart.

   - Swiftly shuffle your feet in place, barely lifting them off the ground.

   - Add arm movements for increased intensity.

2. **Kunoichi Climbers**: (30 seconds)

   - Start in a push-up position.

   - Rapidly draw one knee at a time towards the chest, alternating legs.

   - Keep your back straight and core engaged.

3. **Samurai Squats**: (30 seconds)

   - Stand straight, then drop into a squat.

   - Leap up explosively, arms reaching high.

   - Land softly and repeat immediately.

Rest for 30 seconds between each exercise. Complete this set three times.

Cool Down Tip: End with a brief stretching session to facilitate recovery.

Consistency and Evaluation

Daily practice is key. Aim to incorporate these moves into your routine each day. Track your progress by:

- Counting repetitions: Strive to increase the number each week.

- Timing recovery: Work towards shorter rest periods.

- Monitoring intensity: Push for more explosive and precise movements.

Evaluate your progress every two weeks. Notice improvements in:

- Endurance: You should be able to complete the cycles with less fatigue.

- Strength Gain: Movements will feel easier, allowing for more complete and explosive exercises.

- Agility: Transitions between movements should become smoother and faster.

Remember, mastery takes time. Be patient and persistent; ninja-like agility and strength will develop with consistent effort.

THE ULTIMATE 11-MINUTE SHOULDER SHREDDER

The Key Ideas

- **Time-Efficiency:** Short, intense workouts can be as effective as longer sessions when done correctly.

- **Compound Movements:** Utilize exercises that engage multiple shoulder muscles simultaneously.

- **Progressive Overload:** Continuously challenge your muscles by increasing the intensity of the exercises over time.

- **Mind-Muscle Connection:** Focus on the movement and contraction of the shoulder muscles during the exercises.

- **Recovery:** Allow adequate rest for shoulder muscles to repair and grow.

Practical Implementation

1. **Warm-Up (1 minute):**

   - Arm circles: 15 seconds forward, 15 seconds backward.

   - Shoulder shrugs: 30 seconds.

2. **Workout Sequence (9 minutes):** Perform each exercise for 45 seconds, followed by 15 seconds of rest before moving on to the next.

3. **Dumbbell Shoulder Press:**

4. Stand with feet shoulder-width apart.

5. Push dumbbells from shoulder height to overhead.

   - **Lateral Raises:**

6. Lift dumbbells out to the sides, keeping a slight bend in elbows.

   - **Front Raises:**

7. Raise dumbbells straight in front of you to shoulder height.

   - **Arnold Press:**

8. Start with palms facing you, press dumbbells overhead while rotating to have palms face forward.

   - **Reverse Flyes:**

9. Bend forward slightly, lift dumbbells out to the sides.

   - **Shrugs:**

10. Shrug shoulders towards ears with dumbbells at sides.

    - **Plank with Shoulder Taps:**

11. Tap alternating shoulders while holding a plank position.

    - **Standing Dumbbell Upright Row:**

12. Lift dumbbells close to body with elbows leading.

    - **Pike Push-Ups:**

13. In a pike position, bend elbows to lower head towards ground.

14. **Cool-Down (1 minute):**

   ○ Cross-body shoulder stretch: 30 seconds each side.

Consistency and Evaluation

- **Track Progress:** Record the weight used and the number of repetitions per exercise session.

- **Gradual Increase:** Aim to incrementally increase the weight or the number of repetitions each week.

- **Listen to Your Body:** If you experience any pain, rest and consider consulting a fitness professional.

- **Regular Assessment:** Evaluate your shoulder development and workout intensity every four weeks.

- **Rest and Nutrition:** Prioritize full recovery with adequate sleep and proper nutrition to support muscle growth.

BARRE FITNESS BASICS: BALLET-INSPIRED MOVES IN MINUTES

The Key Ideas

Barre fitness merges ballet, pilates, and yoga to provide a comprehensive workout that focuses on small, isometric movements. The resulting exercises tone the muscles, increase flexibility, and improve balance. While a ballet barre is traditionally used for support, these basics can be adapted for a home setting with sturdy furniture or even a countertop.

- **Muscle Toning Without Bulking**: Barre targets multiple small muscle groups that aren't the focus in typical workouts, promoting a sculpted physique.

- **Flexibility**: Many barre exercises incorporate stretches that enhance flexibility over time.

- **Core Strength**: A strong emphasis on maintaining posture means your core is constantly engaged, leading to better overall stability.

- **Low Impact**: Barre is gentle on the joints, making it accessible for many people, including those with joint concerns or beginners.

Practical Implementation

First, prepare a space with a sturdy chair or counter to use as your makeshift barre. Don comfortable clothing that allows for a full range of motion and bare feet or socks with grip.

1. **Warm-Up (5 Minutes)**:

    ○ Arm circles, shoulder shrugs, and wrist rolls

    ○ Leg swings, knee lifts, and ankle rolls

2. **Leg Work (10 Minutes)**:

    ○ **Plié Squats**: Stand with feet wider than hip-distance, toes turned out. Bend knees and lower your body down, keeping your back straight. Straighten legs to return to the starting position.

    ○ **Leg Lifts**: Stand beside your support and lift one leg at a time to the side, keeping your torso still and tall.

3. **Arm Sculpting (5 Minutes)**:

    ○ **Arm Raises**: Holding small weights or water bottles, start with arms by your side and lift to shoulder height.

    ○ **Bicep Curls**: With your arms in front of you, bend at the elbow to bring the weights toward your shoulders.

4. **Core Integration (5 Minutes)**:

    ○ **Plank**: Hold a plank position from your hands or forearms for 1 minute.

    ○ **Supine Leg Lifts**: Lying on your back, raise and lower your legs while keeping your lower back pressed into the floor.

5. **Cool Down (5 Minutes)**:

    ○ Gentle stretching of all major muscle groups

    ○ Deep breathing to lower your heart rate

Remember to focus on form over speed, paying attention to alignment and breathing.

Consistency and Evaluation

To gain the benefits of barre fitness, aim for consistency. Even short, 10- to 20-minute sessions done several times a week can result in noticeable improvements.

Tracking Progress:

• Note improvements in strength by increased stability during exercises.

• Recognize enhanced flexibility as stretches become easier.

• Record any changes in muscle definition or weight over time.

As you become accustomed to the routines, challenge yourself by adding ankle weights, increasing repetitions, or incorporating more advanced variations of the core exercises. Regular evaluations will help you stay motivated and see the fruits of your dedication to barre fitness.

STEALTHY SCHOOLYARD WORKOUTS: FITNESS AT THE PLAYGROUND

The Key Ideas

Transforming a playground into a fitness hub is an innovative way to get fit. The equipment designed for play doubles as tools for adults seeking to incorporate physical activity into their routine. Here's how:

- **Accessibility**: Playgrounds are widely available and often underutilized during certain hours.

- **Versatility**: The equipment offers various ways to challenge the body, from swing sets to monkey bars.

- **Enjoyment**: An outdoor setting adds a fun element often missing from traditional gyms.

Practical Implementation

To get started, assess the playground for equipment that can support your weight and is safe. Then, integrate these exercises into your routine:

- **Swing Leg Tucks**: Hold the top of a swing, lean back slightly, and use your core to bring your knees towards your chest.

- **Bench Step-Ups**: Use a park bench to perform step-ups to target the legs and glutes.

- **Monkey Bar Pull-Ups**: Grip the bars firmly and pull your body upward, engaging your back and arms.

- **Slide Lunges**: Standing at the base of a slide, place one foot on the slide and lunge, using the slide's incline for added resistance.

Safety Tip: Inspect the equipment for any damage or wet surfaces before use.

Consistency and Evaluation

Set a schedule that works for you, aiming for at least 3 workout sessions per week. Track your progress by:

- Monitoring the number of repetitions and sets.

- Timing how long you can hold a position, like a pull-up.

- Noting improvements in strength or endurance.

Reassessment: Every four weeks, evaluate your progress to tweak and enhance your regimen. Remember, always listen to your body and adjust the intensity to avoid injury.

MINUTE-BY-MINUTE: BUILDING A CUSTOM QUICK WORKOUT

The Key Ideas

• **Time Efficiency:** Maximize the impact of each exercise for a workout that fits into a tight schedule.

• **Personalization:** Adapt the workout to your fitness level, goals, and available equipment.

• **Balance:** Ensure the workout hits all major muscle groups for full-body benefits.

Practical Implementation

1. **Assessment**

   ◦ Determine your current fitness level.

   ◦ Choose exercises that match your goals (strength, endurance, flexibility).

2. **Structure**

   ◦ Prioritize compound movements (exercises that engage multiple muscle groups).

○ Add isolation exercises if time permits, targeting specific muscles.

3. **Sequence**

   ○ Start with a brief dynamic warm-up: jumping jacks, high knees, arm circles.

   ○ Follow with high-intensity resistance training: push-ups, squats, lunges.

   ○ Finish with a quick cool-down: stretching, deep breathing.

4. **Timing**

   ○ Commit to short but intense sessions - 10 to 20 minutes max.

   ○ Use a timer: work for 45 seconds, rest for 15, or any ratio that challenges you.

5. **Variation**

   ○ Change exercises regularly to avoid plateaus.

   ○ Use progression: increase reps, sets, or weights over time.

6. **Preparation**

   ○ Keep your workout gear accessible.

   ○ Designate a specific area for your workouts.

Consistency and Evaluation

- **Routine**

   ○ Slot your quick workout into your daily schedule.

   ○ Aim to be consistent, whether it's every morning or during lunch breaks.

- **Tracking**

  - Keep a log of your workouts: exercises, weights, reps.

  - Monitor your progress and adjust as needed.

- **Feedback**

  - Listen to your body for signs of overtraining or fatigue.

  - Seek variety in your workouts to maintain interest and motivation.

- **Goal Reassessment**

  - Set checkpoints every few weeks to evaluate and reset your fitness goals.

  - Adapt your workout routine to reflect your current objectives.

Let's build a quick workout routine that respects your time constraints while pushing you towards your fitness aspirations. Clear your mind, prep your space, and get ready to transform your body, one minute at a time.

HOTEL ROOM HUSTLE: FULL WORKOUT ON THE GO

The Key Ideas

Your hotel room, far from being a workout wasteland, is ripe with possibilities to help you maintain your fitness schedule. Understanding the principles of bodyweight exercises and utilizing the furnishings creatively can provide you with a comprehensive workout without the need for a gym. Here are the fundamental ideas you'll work with:

- **Leverage What's Available:** Use the bed for incline push-ups, chairs for tricep dips, and towels for resistance exercises.

- **Bodyweight Exercises:** You have all you need for a workout – your body. Exercises like squats, lunges, and planks become your reliable tools.

- **Adaptability Is Key:** Be ready to modify exercises to fit the space and equipment available.

- **Safety First:** Ensure all surfaces are stable and that there's adequate space to avoid injury.

- **Time Management:** Short, intense workouts can be just as effective as longer sessions, especially with time constraints.

Practical Implementation

Begin your workout with a warm-up to get your heart rate up and muscles ready. You can do jumping jacks or high knees in place. Then, move on to a circuit of the following exercises:

1. **Incline Push-Ups** – Using the edge of the bed or a desk.

2. **Chair Dips** – Utilizing the seat of a sturdy chair for tricep dips.

3. **Towel Rows** – A bathroom towel can substitute for resistance bands for back exercises.

4. **Squats and Lunges** – Bodyweight exercises that target the lower body.

5. **Plank Variations** – Forearm, side, and extended arm planks to engage the core.

Perform each exercise for 45 seconds, followed by a 15-second rest. Repeat the circuit 3 to 4 times.

Tips for maximizing the workout:

• Maintain a high intensity, focusing on form and muscle engagement.

• Use slow, controlled movements for increased muscle work.

• Incorporate dynamic movements like jump squats for a cardiovascular boost.

Consistency and Evaluation

To ensure progress:

• **Track Your Workouts**: Note the exercises, reps, and how you felt afterward.

• **Set Clear Goals**: Decide on the frequency of your workouts and set achievable targets.

• **Self-Assess Regularly**: Be honest about the effort you're putting in and the results you're seeing.

It's important to evaluate the effectiveness of your workouts every few weeks. Adjust as necessary, based on progress and any changes in your lifestyle or travel schedule. Remember, the goal is to maintain fitness, not necessarily to break personal records. Consistency will yield results over time.

THE SPEEDY COOL DOWN: PROPER TECHNIQUES FOR A QUICK FINISH

The Key Ideas

Cooling down quickly and efficiently after a workout is just as important as the exercise itself. It's essential for preventing injury and promoting recovery. Here are the most important points to remember:

- Purpose: Understand that cooling down aids in regulating blood flow and reducing muscle stiffness.

- Techniques: Master a few key exercises that facilitate rapid cooling down.

- Timeframe: Keep your cool down brief, around 5-10 minutes, focused on effectiveness rather than duration.

Practical Implementation

Here's how to put these ideas into practice:

1. **Dynamic Stretching:** Start with gentle movement-based stretches that mirror your workout routine. It transitions the body back to a state of rest.

   ◦ Arm circles

- Leg swings

- Torso twists

2. **Static Stretching:** After the initial dynamism, shift to holding stretches for 10-30 seconds that target major muscle groups used.

- Hamstring stretch

- Quad stretch

- Shoulder stretch

3. **Breathing Exercises:** Incorporate deep breathing to lower the heart rate and signal relaxation.

- Inhale for 4 counts

- Hold for 7 counts

- Exhale for 8 counts

4. **Hydrate:** Drink water to replenish fluids and aid in the removal of metabolic waste.

5. **Walk:** Conclude with a brisk walk that gradually slows in pace, helping the cardiovascular system to wind down.

Consistency and Evaluation

To reap the full benefits of a quick cool down, make it a non-negotiable part of your routine:

- **Consistency is Key:** Don't skip this step. Even when pressed for time, a brief cool down prevents injury and aids recovery.

- **Evaluate Effectiveness:** Notice how your body feels. Adjust the duration or techniques based on personal recovery needs.

• **Progress Tracking:** Keep a simple log of your routine, noting any stiffness or soreness.

Always listen to your body and tailor the cool down to personal needs and workout intensity. The right quick cool down routine not only saves time but enhances the overall fitness experience.

CONCLUSION

Wrapping Up Your Fitness Journey with Purpose and Panache

We've sprinted through chapters filled with quick bursts of fitness, each tailored to slot seamlessly into the busy mosaic of your daily life. From the *7-Minute Full Body Blast* to the *Speedy Cool Down*, this book has been your trusty sidekick in weaving movement, strength, and vitality into the fabric of your time-starved schedule.

The Fitness Montage of Your Life

Imagine your exercise routine as a personal highlight reel—a montage of you conquering the *Ultimate Push-Up Challenge*, stretching into the day with a *Morning Quick-Start*, or exuding focus through a *Yoga Flow for Serenity*. Every chapter has been a scene in this montage, starring you as the hero who manages time like a caped crusader.

Take-Aways from Each Fitness Episode

- **HIIT for Busy Bees**: Remember, ten minutes committed wholeheartedly to an intense workout can trump a half-hearted hour.

- **Lunch Break Power Walk & Tone-Up**: Convert what's usually downtime into a potent mix of cardio and strength, blending a brisk walk with discrete toning exercises.

- **5-Minute Deskercise**: Never underestimate the power of the small. Five minutes of office-friendly moves keep the sedentary blues at bay.

- **Plyometric Power**: Explosiveness isn't just for athletes. Incorporating rapid movements can significantly enhance your muscle power.

- **Tabata Torch**: Blink and you'll miss it; this 4-minute fat-burning blitz is proof that fitness feats need not be time leeches.

Embedding Fitness into Everyday Life

- **Supermarket Shape-Up**: Who knew aisle five could double as your track, or that the frozen foods section offers the perfect spot for some quick squats?

- **Commute Cycle**: Reimagine your daily commute as an opportunity for interval training. Pedal your way to better health.

- **TV Time Toning**: Binge fitness while you binge-watch. Those commercial breaks are gold mines for some muscle sculpting.

Embracing Fitness as a Lifelong Companion

You've likely realized by now that fitness is less about monumental daily efforts and more about the consistency of small, deliberate actions. Whether you're performing isometric exercises on the restroom sink or practicing speed tai chi stretches while your coffee brews, you're cultivating a habit that thrives on regularity rather than volume.

The Pro Tips to Keep in Your Back Pocket

1. **Prioritize Form Over Speed**: Even when time is sparse, poor form can lead to injury and diminish the effectiveness of your workouts.

2. **Mix and Match**: Keep your body guessing and your mind engaged by combining chapters. Stairwell workouts today, kettlebell combat tomorrow?

3. **Stay Equipped**: Keep resistance bands, a jump rope, or a set of dumbbells within reach. Little fitness allies can make a big difference.

The Long Run: Keeping the Momentum Going

The journey doesn't end here. As you turn the final page of this book, consider it not as a conclusion, but rather a bookmark in your lifelong adventure in fitness. Reflect on the growth you've experienced and the habits you've nurtured.

Foster Resilience and Flexibility

Life, ever unpredictable, will surely throw curveballs that disrupt your newly-formed fitness cadence. Embrace this uncertainty and adjust on the fly. Substitute stretches when you can't manage a full workout, or mentally rehearse your routine to keep your mind in the game.

Celebrate Your Victories, No Matter the Size

From mastering the *Dynamic Warm-Ups* to confidently executing the *Speed Endurance Drills*, each milestone is a triumph worth celebrating. Revel in these moments—they are the fuel that will propel you onward.

Spread the Fitness Cheer

Share your journey. Become the advocate of quick workouts among friends, family, and colleagues. Illustrate through your actions how seamlessly fitness can intertwine with a bustling life.

And, as you forge ahead, remember: *Fitness for the Time-Pressed* isn't just a series of workouts; it's a mindset, an ethos that champions the truth that there is always time for health, and that every minute, when lived fully, counts.

Stay nimble, be tenacious, and keep the chapters of this book not just on your shelf but in your heart as you continue to write your own story of personal well-being.

Now, get out there and make each minute magnificent!